Radiology of Positioning for Technician

SECOND EDITION

Prof. O.P. Sharma
MD, PhD, FAMS
Retd. Professor and Head
Department of Radiology
Institute of Medical Sciences
Banaras Hindu University
Varanasi
Uttar Pradesh

PEEPEE
PUBLISHERS AND DISTRIBUTORS (P) LTD.

Radiology of Positioning for Technician

Published by
Pawaninder P. Vij and Anupam Vij
Peepee Publishers and Distributors (P) Ltd.
Head Office: 160, Shakti Vihar, Pitam Pura
Delhi-110 034 (India)

Correspondence Address:
7/31, First Floor, Ansari Road, Daryaganj
New Delhi-110 002 (India)
Ph: 41512412, 23246245, 9811156083
e-mail: peepee160@yahoo.co.in
e-mail: peepee160@rediffmail.com
e-mail: peepee160@gmail.com
www.peepeepub.com

First Edition: **2007**
Second Edition: 2018

ISBN: 978-81-8445-239-6

Preface to the Second Edition

I am pleased to introduce the second edition of my book entitled **"Radiology of Positioning for Technician"** in current year (2018) after a gap of almost ten years of its first edition published by Peepee Publishers and Distributors (P) Ltd., New Delhi.

This second edition will provide you much more detail about special procedure in conventional radiology with help of black / white machine picture and its result.

Some new chapters on positron-emission-tomography CT Scan (PET–CT), B.M.D. (Bone densitometry) and digital subtraction angiography have been added.

Now-a-days C.T. Scan and its allied development has contributed much more detail on PET–CT, a new vista for those student pursuing CT–technician course which provides the job opportunity to great extent than before hence this edition will prove worthy for new generation student.

I believe, the 2nd edition of this book will be a boon to student pursuing technician course in Radiodiagnosis particularly CT Scan and PET–CT Scan and to some extent to diploma and Degree course of medical student as well.

Prof. O. P. Sharma

Acknowledgements

I am extremely thankful to Mr. Pawaninder P. Vij, Director M/s. Peepee Publishers and Distributors (P) Ltd., New Delhi for publishing the second edition of **Radiology of Positioning for Technician**. I hope, all the readers will be benefited with this book.

Mr. Bhupendra Bahadur Prajapati for his help in preparing the advance script of this book in present form.

Prof. O. P. Sharma

Contents

1. **General Considerations: Applied Physics** 1
   - Introduction...1
   - X-ray Films...21
   - Acquisition of Radiograph...28
   - Dark-Room Chemistry...29
   - Dark-Room Artefacts...32
   - Maximum Permissible Dose (MPD)...33
2. **Radiographic Positioning** 35
   - Head and Neck...43
   - Spine or Vertebral Column...57
   - Chest...66
   - Heart and Great Vessels...73
   - View for Foreign Body Esophagus and Left Atrial Enlargement...76
   - Diaphragm...77
   - Abdomen...78
   - Urinary Tract and Retroperitoneal Structures...81
   - Anteroposterior (for Pregnancy) View...82
   - Anteroposterior View for Liver...82
   - Anteroposterior View for Spleen...82
   - Upper Extremity...83
   - Lower Extremity...95
   - Pelvis...110

3. **Radiological Procedures Including Contrast Media** 121
   - Intravascular Contrast Media...126
   - Gastrointestinal Tract...141
4. **Ultrasonography** 205
5. **Computed Tomography** 218
   - Use or Indications of CT Scanning...229
   - How Do I Prepare the Patient?...230
   - How Does the Equipment Look Like?...231
6. **PET–CT** 235
7. **Magnetic Resonance Imaging** 240
8. **Mammography** 259
9. **Bone Density Measurement in Osteoporosis and Osteopenia on DEXA Machine** 269
10. **Digital Subtraction Angiography** 274
11. **Harmful Effects of Radiation** 278
    - Radiation Measurements and Its Biological Effects...279
    - Radiation Protection...297
    - Unit for Study of Radiation...319

Index 323

1

General Considerations: Applied Physics

INTRODUCTION

X-Rays

Late in 1895, Wilhelm Conrad Roentgen, while observing a Crooke's vacuum tube operated at high voltage, noticed that a piece of barium platinocyanide lying several feet away from the end of tube glowed in the dark. He quickly realized that the fluorescence (glowing in the dark) of the barium platinocyanide, must have been produced by invisible radiation coming from the tube. Roentgen then placed his hand between the tube and a sheet of cardboard coated with barium platinocyanide, his hand bone was seen as image. Roentgen gave the name **'X-ray'** to this invisible penetrating radiation and finally the rays was termed as Roentgen rays.

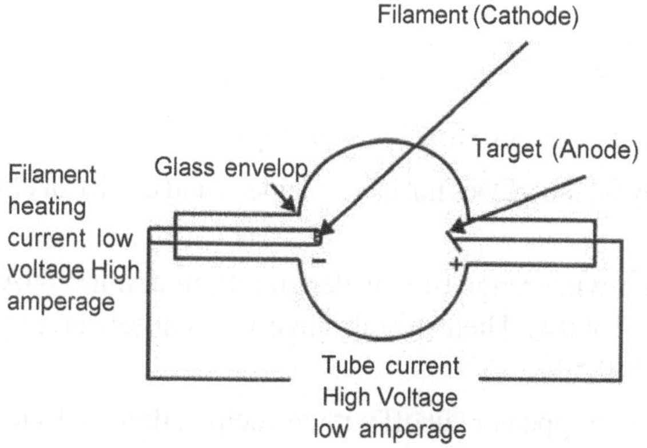

Fig. 1.1: X-ray tube

Roentgen rays are a type of electromagnetic wave travelling at a speed as high as 1,86,000 miles per second in a vacuum. These rays arise whenever a stream of fast moving electrons are suddenly slowed down or stopped by placing something in their way. A man made device in which X-ray or roentgen rays are produced is called an X-ray or roentgen tube.

When a stream of electrons strikes at the tube target (Anode with a positive charge), X-rays are produced by the following two main processes:

1. Radiation.
2. Characteristic radiation.

Anode target is made up of tunsten having high melting point and high atomic number. It has a melting point of 3370°C and an atomic number of 74. The vapour pressure of tungsten at high temperature is relatively low (at temperatures above 1650°C, 3000 °F) and the highest tensile strength. The vacuum within the tube is thus more likely to be preserved and protected. To facilitate the dissipation of heat from the anode target, tungsten plate is embedded in a block of copper having low melting point, which is a better conductor of heat and helps to maintain the temperature of tungsten low. This copper block is inturn cooled by the high-tension transformer oil surrounding the X-ray tube and finally the atmospheric air cools the oil. The electron beam striking at the Tungsten target is termed as the **focal spot**.

Properties of X-rays

1. They are highly penetrating invisible rays.
2. Electrically neutral–Does not have magnetic and electrical effect on them.
3. Occurs in a wide range of wavelengths from about 0.04Å to more than 1000Å. Their useful range in roentgenography is about 0.1Å-0.5Å.
4. They can be stopped or cut off with the help of thin lead sheets. (Cut off the X-rays depends upon the penetrating power of the X-rays and the thickness of the lead sheet).

5. Roentgen rays are heterogeneous in nature and are of different wavelengths.
6. Emerges from the tube in straight line (Can be produced efficiently in a device by suddenly slowing down of fast moving electrons).
7. Their intensity decreases with the amount of matter and with increase in the distance between the source and the object.
8. Can travel at a speed of light.
9. It can ionize matter, as they have ability to remove orbital electrons from atoms.
10. It can cause fluorescence effect (Invisible X-rays can be converted into visible light).
11. It cannot be focused by a lens.
12. It effects photographic film and can produce latent image (Invisible image).
13. It can produce chemical and biological changes in matter.
14. Can produce secondary and scattered radiation.

Hard X-ray

It has relatively high frequency, short wavelength, high penetrating power and little absorption in the skin as compared with in interior of body. It can be produced by using:

- Higher kilo voltage.
- Filters such as aluminium or copper.
- Tube target of high atomic number.

Filters: They are employed between the patient and the X-ray tube (on the X-ray tube assembly) to alter the quality of a beam of X-rays. They also reduce the total intensity of the beam. A simple filter consists of a thin sheet of material in which the attenuation increases rapidly with decrease in photon energy (as the energies commonly used in radiology) so that there is much greater attenuation of the low photon energy (long wavelength) radiation than of the high photon energy (short wavelength) radiation in the beam. The shape of the spectrum is therefore altered.

The filtered beam is described as harder (i.e., more penetrating) than the unfiltered beam because it contains a higher proportion of high photon energy radiation, which are more penetrating. In diagnostic X-rays the material most often chosen is aluminium.

Soft X-ray

It has relatively low frequency with long wavelength as compared to hard rays. They have low penetrating power. Therefore has greater absorption in skin. They may be followed by:

- Lower kilo voltage.
- Unfiltered X-rays.
- Target used for X-ray generation is of low atomic number.

  Basically there is one anode and one cathode. The cathode is also termed as filament.
- A heated cathode filament act as the source of thermionic emission of electron. The rate of emission increases with the temperature of the filament, which depends on the filament current measured in amperes (mAs).
- If no kilovoltage is applied, the emitted electrons remain near the filament as an electron cloud or space charge.
- If a kilovoltage is applied between Cathode (–) and Anode (+), the electron are driven over to the anode by the large potential difference. The average speed of the electrons increases as the kilovoltage is increased. The flow of electrons across the gap between the cathode and anode constitutes the tube current, measured in milliamperes (ma).
- If the electron speed is high enough, X-rays are produced due to striking of the electrons on the anode target. The energy is being converted to heat (99.8%) and X-ray are only (0.2%).

The cathode and the anode are sealed in a tube made up of Pyrax glass, in which high vacuum has been produced and air is evacuated out of glass and metal by baking process called as degassing. The entire tube is immersed in insulating oil (High-tension transformer oil–insulator and coolant) within a suitable metal housing.

The cathode filament in most diagnostic tube measures about 0.2 cm in diameter and 1 cm or less in length. The filament is backed by a negatively charged concave molybdenum cup (Cathode focussing cup) which confines the electrons to a narrow beam and focuses them on a small part on tungsten target known as the focal spot, which acts as a source of X-rays.

As the tube gets older, a progressively lower filament current setting is required for a desired tube milliamperage.

Mobile X-ray equipments have a single filament; modern diagnostic X-ray tubes are provided with two filaments mounted side by side. One is smaller than the other is. A switch is provided in the control equipment to select one or the other filament as the source of electron. These produce focal spots of two different sizes on the target "double focus tube", actually it is a double filament tube.

X-ray tube anode are of two types:

- Stationary Anode.
- Rotating Anode.

Stationary Anode

Stationary X-ray tubes are used in the small portable units, where small amount of X-ray exposures are given for a small interval of time. The stationary anodes have a small focal area and has a shorter life than that of the rotating anodes due to the striking of the electrons onto the target a small area the anode smooth surface is spoiled and small pits are produced. On a defective anode, the amount of scattering increase and the primary radiations are reduced to a considerable amount.

The filament of the cathode is made up of fine tungsten wire coiled to form a small helix or vertical spiral. Tungsten has a high melting point and has reasonably high electron emission at a given temperature, and has good mechanical strength and physical properties, which allow it to be drawn into fine wire and wound into a spiral shape. The tendency of tungsten is to vaporize at high temperature is relatively low, and so the filament has a reasonably long life.

Inside the cathode-focussing cup, a small hole is made, so that one end of the heated filament pass through it by insulation and in no way it is in contact with the cathode-focussing cup. Other end of the filament is grounded (in contact) with the cathode focussing cup.

The anode of the X-ray tube is a solid cylindrical copper block with its inner end cut to present a sloping flat circular face towards the cathode. The face being at about 18^{0} to 20^{0} . This anode block passes through one end of the tube to the exterior where it can be connected by means of a high-tension cable to the positive side of the high-tension supply, so that anode go positive with respect to the negative cathode.

The anode target is a small plate of tungsten two to three millimeters thick, which is inset into the copper and has its outer surface level with the angled face of the anode. The plate may be rectangular or square, a size of about 1 cm $\times$ 0.5 cm being typical and the electrons are focused to bombard at a focal area close to its center. This is termed as focal spot and act as a source of x-radiation.

The target is backed by the massive copper anode block, because of the higher specific heat of copper combined with the large mass of metal used, results in the anode having a much greater thermal capacity than if it were all tungsten. As a result, the temperature rise for a given number of calories absorbed is smaller. The good thermal conductivity of copper permits the heat to be conducted rapidly away to the exterior of the tube. The provision for supporting the tube in a metal shield does dissipating heat from the exterior end of the anode filled with high tension transformer oil, the oil act as both coolant and electrical insulation. Most stationary anodes have effective focuses of 2 mm and 4 mm.

Rotating Anode

The anode of the X-ray tube is a disc of solid tungsten, which **rotates at a speed of about 3,000 revolutions to 9000 revolutions per minute** during the exposure period. The stem of the disc is made up of molybdenum having a melting point of 2600°C. The disc has a **beveled edge, the angle of the bevel to a vertical being usually about 16.5°**. This complete beveled edge act as a focal spot for the entire period of the exposure. The induction motor helps the anode to rotate.

The main features of a rotating anode tube is the **vacuum envelope made up of heat resistant borosilicate glass**. The Cathode cup and the filament are off set from the longitudinal axis of the tube, and are positioned opposite the target track, which is near the periphery of the anode disc.

The three important factors of the rotating anode tube are as follows:

1. The anode rotates on ball bearings, which must absorb very little heat from the tungsten disc, since otherwise their is smooth bearing properties will deteriorate.
2. Part of the anode system is the rotor of an induction motor and must have suitable electric and magnetic properties.
3. The rotation of the anode must be perfectly balanced, so that the disc is free of vibrations, which would disturb the position of the target area, and thus cause image blur as well as adding undue wear to the ball bearings.

The anode disc which must rotates during radiographic exposures is connected by stem(s) made up of molybdenum, which is a hard white metal with atomic number as 42, melting point is about 2600°C and atomic mass about half that of tungsten.

Radiographic Quality

It denotes visibility and sharpness of the image with structural details.

Four factors are responsible for radiographic quality:

a. Definition.

b. Density.

c. Contrast.

d. Distortion.

Definition: Definition is a sharpness of structure lines or minute details in a roentgenogram. Good definition permits the detection of minimal changes in the structure, i.e., the abruptness of boundary between the two structures.

Resolution: Resolution is the ability of an imaging system to produce separate images of closely spaced objects.

Note: The two entities described above though separate but are governed by similar factors. These two when recorded, are known as objective. When it is seen by a radiologist, is subjective sharpness/resolution/definition.

Factors governing definition and resolution:

1. **Geometric factors:** The geometric factors are related with arrangement in space of X-ray beam, object to be radiographed and recording medium.

   These are:

   - *Size of effective focus:* With a smaller focal spot the sharpness of the radiograph will increase.
   - *Focus-film distance (FFD):* It controls magnification and image unsharpness as the distance is increased, the effect is similar to a decrease in focal spot size.
   - *Object-film distance (OFD):* If the FFD remains unchanged and only the OFD is altered then by application of geometric principles we find that a decreased in the OFD decreases the penumbra (scattered) thereby enhance the definition. By increasing the OFD, the magnification of the image will also be increased, thereby decreasing the sharpness of the film image.
   - *Alignment of object vis-a-vis the film and the beam:* The object should be kept parallel to the film in outline and shape.

If not placed paralleled to the film the object will be foreshortened. If oblique rays were used, distortion of the image would be produced.

2. **Motion unsharpness:** It can be caused due to the movement of the patient of the cassette or X-ray tube during exposure.
3. **Object unsharpness:** Objects exposed are not made perfect and the exposure is given according to the centre of the object. Overall image unsharpness can be calculated on the entire film or the object exposed.
4. **Film unsharpness.**
5. **Parallax unsharpness:** Double coated X-ray films used can produce parallax type of unsharpness, as the image is formed on both sides in the emulsion layer.
6. **Screen unsharpness:** The sharpness of the fluorescent image is reduced as the speed of the screen increases. The film should be in close contact with intensifying screen. Any fuzziness on the processed film image indicates a lack of screen film contact.
7. **Total unsharpness.**

Density

The amount of darkening of an X-ray film or of a certain area on the film is called radiographic density. A diagnostic radiograph usually has densities varying from about 0.4 in lightest areas to 3.0 in the darkest area.

$$\text{Density (D)} = \text{Log}\ \frac{I_0}{I_1}$$

Where I_0 = Intensity of incidence light

I_1 = Intensity of transmitted light.

The factors affecting the contrast:

1. *Radiation Quality or Penetrability (KVP)*—Increasing KV increases the penetrability of primary radiation hence decreasing the contrast. Also this occurs because of increased scattered

radiation but this can be overcome by the use of grid (Grid eliminates/reduces the amount of scattered radiation).

2. *Object*—Thickness of tissue is important for X-ray attenuation; it also depends upon the nature of organ exposed to X-ray, which is important. Same thickness of tooth enamel will attenuate X-ray more than bone, which in turn is more than an osteoporosed bone. Due to this reason, we use contrast media whenever possible to increase the subject contrast.
3. *Use of Screen*—Intensifying screen increases the average gradient or slope of a film hence increasing contrast. It basically affects the radiographic contrast.
4. *Film Processing Technique*—Time and temperature of development, composition of developing chemicals and their strength and method of developing process (whether automatic or manual) affects the contrast of the film.
5. *Filtration*—Filter is used to remove unwanted, unhealthy and radiographically useless X-ray photon from the beam. This process increases the contrast.

   An ideal filter material should have the following prerequisites:

   a. In order to discriminate against low energy photons, the absorption must have photoelectric effect.
   b. The absorbing material should not have an absorption edge near the energy of desirable photons.
   c. The thickness of material should be very less, e.g., nearly ¼ mm or less.

   Looking into these requirements, the good materials are lead, tin, copper, aluminium or the mixed compound filter.

6. *Fogging*—Causes reduction in the contrast of an X-ray film. Fog is the visual effect produced by the development of those silver halides crystal, which are not exposed or less, exposed to X-ray thus forming unwanted image on an X-ray film.
7. *Scattered Radiation*—Reduces contrast by fogging effect mainly on the lighter areas of films. Primary beam is the group of rectilinear X-rays emitted by the target metal as its

characteristics radiation when electrons strike its atoms. When passed through an object, some of these rays are absorbed, while others are scattered and transmitted. The scattered radiation reach the film and lead to fogging.

Scattered radiation increased by:

1. An increase in area of radiation field.
2. An increase in thickness of area irradiated.
3. An increase in density of tissue irradiated.
4. An increase in tube potential.
5. A decrease in OFD.

Speed of a film is only a relative value that shows how much exposure is required to produce a density of one.

$$\text{Speed} = \frac{100}{\text{MR to produce density 1}}$$

Factors Affecting Density

1. **K.V.:** Any increase in KV, increases the density. 15% increase in KV leads to doubling of exposure. But very high exposure increase the fogging effect.
2. **mA (Tube Current):** It is number of electrons running from cathode to anode per second. Its increase leads to proportionate increase in amount of X-rays (mR). Density changes with changes in tube current (mA).
3. **Time of Exposure:** According to reciprocity law, it is the change in mAs that changes the exposure, increasing one and decreasing the other, may have no effect. Increased mAs increases the exposure.
4. **Distance:** Increasing the distance, decreases the density as smaller number of rays, that are actually diverging, fall on a unit area of film. Also because the density of radiation falls as distance increases by inverse square law.

$$I \propto \frac{1}{d^2}$$

5. *Thickness and Nature of Part:* Although contrast may not be changed but the density, decreases with increase in object thickness.

Contrast of the Film

Contrast of a radiographic image on film is defined as the difference in optical densities of two points on the same film (i.e., light and dark area). Minimum of 0.02 contrast must be present for two object to be delineated separately. Another way to define is that contrast is the straight portion of the characteristic curve.

Factors affecting Contrast could be:

(i) **Subject Contrast:** It is the result of differences in absorption of radiation by the part under examination. Factors which effect subject contrast are:

(a) *Subject Itself:* Subject contrast depends on the thickness, density and atomic number of the part being X-rayed. Greater the difference in the X-ray attenuation by the part being X-rayed, greater will be the subject contrast. If the difference in attenuation is small then in order to achieve a higher contrast the thickness of the subject must be large.

(b) *Radiation Quality:* As discussed earlier the KVP determines the penetrating power of the X-ray beam. If the KVP selected is too low, almost all the X-rays are attenuated by patient and nothing reaches the film. Hence KVP selected has a great effect on subject contrast. Low KVP will produce high contrast, provided the KVP is high enough to penetrate the part being examined adequately.

As a general rule, low KVP gives high subject contrast. This is often called short scale contrast because everything is black or white on the film with fewer shades in between. High KVP gives lower subject contrast, called long scale contrast, of shades of grey in between the lightest and darkest portion of the image.

(c) *Scatter and Fog:* The effect of fog and scatter is to reduce radiographic contrast and as such undesirable.

Scatter radiation increases with part thickness, field size and energy of X-ray beam (higher KVP).

Scatter radiation can be minimized by collimation of X-ray beam and use of grids or air gaps.

Scatter radiation that reaches the X-ray film or film screen combination produces unwanted density or image blurr.

(ii) **Film Contrast:** Radiographic contrast also depends on the film recording system, a designation which includes film and processing with or without screen.

(a) *Film:* The important property of films which we wish to use in radiography is the ability of X-ray radiation to produce a visible pattern of varying depths of blackness in the film which is known as density. The relationship between density and exposure is contained in what is known as characteristic curve of film. The actual shape of the curve is controlled by the detailed way the film was made, stored and processed.

(b) *Film Exposure:* An underexposed radiograph will have poor contrast and therefore the final quality of the film is poor.

(c) *Film Processing:* It is one of the most important factors which affect the film contrast.

(i) *Development:* Is a chemical process, the purpose of which is to render visible the latent image which is formed in the emulsion of film during exposure.

It is important to see that the developer used is of correct composition, temperature and pH. The activity of the developer should be checked and replenishment should be carried out as and when the activity of the developer is reduced.

The chemical composition, temperature, the time for which developer is allowed to act and the degree of agitation of film in the solution during development affects the film density and hence quality. Increase in reducing power of the chemical (fresh chemical), increase in time and temperature increases film density. Temperature and time can be used to compensate for each other, and for a typical situation the followed pair of value will produce the same degree of development.

75° F - 2.5 min. 65° F - 5 min.

In manual processing the blackening should be regularly checked during developing and the operator should decide when the development process needs to be stopped. The film under process should be removed out of the developing chemical on achievement of the desired density and shifted to rinser. The overlong examination of the films during the developing process in presence of dark room lights often gives rise to fog formation. This should be borne in mind to process the film in the lowest intensity of light and in the shortest possible time.

(ii) *Fixing:* Before transferring the developed film into fixer solution for fixing of image, it should be rinsed properly in water to prevent developer which accompany film from entering fixer. It should be noted that fixer should be of correct composition and is changed whenever required.

(iii) *Final Rinsing:* It is done with free flow of water to remove all fixing bath chemicals. This final rinsing takes place in running water. The time for final rinsing depends on temperature of water.

Temperature of Water	Duration of Rinsing
41 - 54° F	30 min.
55 - 77° F	20 min.
78 - 88° F	15 min.
Over 88° F	10 min.

(iv) *Drying:* Before placing the film in dryer, it should be left for two minutes in a wetting agent. This reduces the surface tension of water, dampens the entire surface uniformly and the film can thus be dried more quickly and without any risk of forming spots. Before shifting the film to drier. It should be kept hanging for sometime to drain of water.

Method of Reducing Scattered Radiation

A. Reducing Production of Scattered Radiation

a. *Reducing the beam size:* By using beam restricting devices (cones, diaphragm, collimators etc.) these reduces the radiation dose to patient and penumbra effect.

b. *Compression:* Pushes away excess compressible tissue from the field.

c. *Appropriate use of KV:* Increase in KV, increases the scattered radiation by increasing compton effect and number of forward moving photons therefore KVP should be kept to reasonably low-level. By using low Kvp, it increases the radiation absorption dose to the patient in decreasing the radiation quality.

B. Reduction of Scattered Radiation Reaching the Film:

a. Use of grid.

b. Metal backing of cassette.

c. Filters:

- Metallic filter.
- Air gap.

d. Reduction of effect of scattered radiation on film and by use of screens which are acting as filter and are more sensitive to hardening primary photon—selectively intensity enhancement.

Distortion: Image produced on a radiograph is not the exact representation of the anatomic part being imaged but differs from it, in varying degree of shape and size. Such misrepresentation of the size and shape of an object is called "Distortion".

Radiographic image can be distorted in size and shape.

(i) *Size Distortion (Magnification):* When an object is held between the source of light and a white surface, the size of the shadow enlarges as the object is moved nearer to the light and shrinks as it is moved closer to white surface. This is due to divergence of rays in the beam. The shorter the distance between the object and source of light the greater is the magnification. Magnification or size distortion can be decreased by either reducing OFD or increasing FFD.

(ii) *Shape Distortion:* It is caused by improper alignment of object, with relation to tube and film. The object merely gets oblique in direction.

Heel effect: Is the variation in exposure rate with the angle of emission of radiation from focus and film focus distance. The radiation is greatest at cathode end and least at anode end. This can be taken advantage of by placing thicker part towards cathode end and so on to get a uniform image.

Grid: Grid is a device made up of parallel lead strip separated by radiolucent material [of thickness = (d) and separated by interspace material of thickness = D]. Its chief function is to reduce scattered radiation and to increase the contrast of the film.

There are two basic disadvantages of using grids:

1. Presence of grid lines on finished radiographic image.
2. By using grid, it increases the amount of Kvp to be used during exposure to the patient.

The grid reduces the scattered radiation to the extent of 90% but also removes the primary radiation by 10-15% depending on the grid ratio (h/d–It is the ratio between the height of lead strip and the distance between two lead strips) and hence are the grid lines formed. Grid lines can be overcome by blurring them by moving the grid continously during exposure.

$$\text{The contrast improvement factor (k)} = \frac{\text{Contrast with grid}}{\text{Contrast without grid}}$$

Grid Ratio (γ):

$$\gamma = h/D$$

h = height of strips.

D = interspace between the lead strips.

Higher the ratio, more is the clean up and better is the contrast. The straighter rays can only penetrate the high ratio grid. Usually $\gamma = 5\text{-}12$, never > 16.

$$\text{Grid Factor: } \frac{\text{Exposure needed with grid}}{\text{Exposure needed without grid}} = \text{usually 2-6}$$

The functional factor (k) depend on KV, thickness of object and field size, so have a variable and limited interpretative values.

Types of Grids

Linear Grid (Parallel or Unfocused Grid)—The lead strips are parallel to each other in their longitudinal axis. Most X-ray tables are equipped with such linear grids. Their major advantage is that they allow us to angle the X-ray tube along the length of the grid (longitudinal axis) without loss of primary radiation from grid "cut off". In this case the angulation of the X-ray tube cannot be given in crosswise direction. If the rays are not exactly parallel to the grid lines then the rays are prevented from reaching the film. This is the disadvantage of using a linear grid.

Focused Grid—A focused grid is made up of lead strips that are angled slightly so that they focus in shape and joins in space at single line or point. A focused grid may be either linear or crossed, because the focusing refers to the cross-sectional plane of the lead strips. Most grids are focused. Linear focused grids converges at a line in space called the convergent line. This convergent line clearly explains that the X-ray tube should be operated from this line during exposure to avoid primary radiation from grid cut-off with the acceptable focus to film distance. Similarly, crossed grids coverage at a point in space called the convergent point (One convergent line for the each superimposed linear grid and both these convergent lines are intersecting at an imaginary point in space called convergent point). The focal distance is the perpendicular distance between the grid and the convergent line or point. In practice, grids have a focusing range that indicates the distance within which the grid can be used without a significant loss of primary radiation.

The focusing range is fairly wide for a low ratio grid and narrow for a high ratio grid. A 5:1 grid is focused at 40" FFD and works at a focusing range of approx. 28 to 72 inches, while 16:1 grid focused is focussed at 40" and works at a focusing range of only 32 to 42 inches. Manufacturers indicate focal ranges on the top of grids. A parallel grid is one in which the lead strips are parallel when viewed in cross-section. They are focused at infinity, so that do not have a convergent line. These grids can only be used effectively with either very small X-ray fields or long target grid distances. They are frequently used in fluoroscopic spot film devices, but otherwise have little use in modern radiology.

Pseudo-focused Grid—In this grid, the height of peripheral lines is less therefore reducing the grid ratio peripherally. This grid, though, easy to manufacture, has an overall efficiency similar to focused grid.

Crossed Grid—A crossed grid is made up of two superimposed linear grid (One is lengthwise and the other in the crosswise directions) that have the same focusing distance. The grid ratio of crossed grids is equal to the some of the ratios of the two linear grids. A crossed grid made up of two 5:1 linear grids will have a grid ratio of 10:1 ratio. Crossed grids cannot be used with oblique techniques requiring angulations of the X-ray tube and this is their biggest disadvantage of this type.

Moving Grid—Moving grids are fixed below the X-ray table and above the bucky. With the help of electrical motor it is made to move back and forth continuously. But, in case of casualty radiography and in case of portable X-rays where the patient cannot be shifted on to the X-ray table than in such cases stationary grids are employed and a compromise is made with the radiographic quality. Stationary grids have the same structure as that of the moving grid, but they donot move during the exposure. There are chances of getting grid cut-off image due to not properly placing of the stationary grids (Tilting and not perpendicular to X-ray beam, not properly focussed, FFD not proper etc.).

Characteristic Curve

It is also called as H.D. curve or Sensitometric curve.

It shows the relation of density change (contrast) to change in exposure (in Log scale).

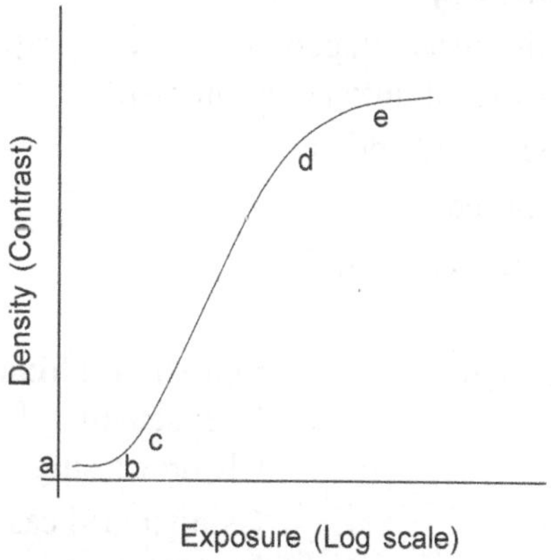

Fig. 1.2

a-b or fog level: It is basal density, inherent to a film for a good film, this is minimal.

c-d or straight line: Density in this region is uniformly proportional to exposure. This is the most radiographically relevant area. Its slope is known as Gamma (γ), measures maximum density difference chosen from two exposures.

γ is entirely a film's inherent property. It is usually 4.

$$\gamma = \frac{D_2 - D_1}{LogE_2 - LogE_1}$$

$$\text{or } \gamma \left(\text{Log} \frac{E_2}{E_1}\right) = D_2 - D_1$$

$$\text{Hence C} = \gamma \left(\text{Log} \frac{E_2}{E_1}\right)$$

C-D is known as "Region of correct exposure". γ can be increased by increase in developer concentration, time, temperature and agitation.

Toe and shoulder area (bc and de): Are areas of low slope where large change in exposure is required to cause change in density.

Grid: Further Reading

1. If grid is not properly placed while radiography is being performed it may result into poor contrast.
2. It may be placed up side down.
3. It may be off centred.
4. It may produce grid errors i.e.

   Moire effect.

   Zebra pattern : Caused by : Similar grid frequency to laser scanning frequency in CR processing.

   : Using a grid cassette in the bucky tray.

   : Corrected by : Selecting a high grid frequency

   Use a moving grid mechanism.

   Do not use two grid.

Grid Selection:

Less than 90 Kvp - 8:1 grid ratio is satisfactory.

More than 90 Kvp - more 8:1 grid ratio should be used.

As grid ratio increases, transmission of scatter radiation decreases faster than transmission of primary radiation therefore clear up of scattered radiation increases.

Grid	Clinical Consideration in Grid selection			Comment
	Degree of scatter removal	Off-centre latitude	KVP	
5:1	+	Very Wide	Up to 80	Low cost, easy to use.
6:1	+	Very Wide	Up to 80	Low cost, mobile radiography.
8:1 - 10:1	+/+++	Wide	Up to 100	General stationary examinations.
12:1	++++	Narrow	Over 110	Precise centering, usually fixed mount.
16:1	+++++	Narrow	Over 110	Precise centering, usually fixed mounts

X-RAY FILMS

An X-ray film has following layers:

Base—.18 mm thick polyester plastic or cellulose triacetate sheet tinted in blue. By virtue of it being non-explosive and non-inflammable, the modern film is known as a "safety film" (e.g. polyester base-polyethylene terephthelate). This is the thickest layer but most transparent and does not take up any visible pattern. Its function is just to support the emulsion. The base expands on processing in a direction perpendicular to itself and contracts later on thereby maintaining the position of image.

Emulsion—Consists of numerous flat, triangular particles of Ag Br (Silver bromide) and other silver halides (AgI) suspended in gelatin, spread uniform and parallel to the base. The layer of emulsion is 1/1000 inch thick and is present on both sides and hence these films are known as double coated or deputized films. While preparing, only the gelatin is treated with mustard oil to add traces of sulphur as impurities (called as Ripening). This and other impurities are actually responsible for the latent image. This is light sensitive and most delicate layer of film which once applied, should be protected from light and tapering.

A layer of solvent for base and gelatin which acts as adhesive. A gelatin layer for protection of emulsion known as supercoating. This film is a very delicate structure and should be handled with utmost care against tapering and light. It is important to carry it in a sturdy holder known as a CASSETTE or CARDBOARD HOLDER.

Latitude and Sensitivity (SPEED) are basic emulsion characteristics. Sensitivity is the ability of an emulsion to respond to radiation or in other words, a fat emulsion will respond to even a little exposure.

Latitude on the other hand describes how well a picture of an object will be depicted or in scientific terms the ability of an emulsion to display an image with reasonably a long range of tones, i.e., long scale contrast. This aspect of latitude is known as long tonal range. There is another aspect known as Permissible Margin of Error in exposures, this is its ability to allow a reasonable error in exposure without seriously tapering the radiographic quality.

Latitude of the X-ray film refers to the range of relative exposure (mAs) that will produce density within the accepted range for diagnostic radiology (usually considered to be density between 0.25 and 2.0).

$$\text{Speed} = \frac{100}{\text{MR to form density 1}}$$

Depends on crystal number and size

$$\gamma \propto \frac{1}{\text{Speed}}$$

OR

$$\gamma \propto \frac{1}{\text{Latitude}}$$

Types of Films

1. **Screen film**—Films exposed with the use of intensifying screens placed in the cassettes.
2. **Non screen film or Direct exposure film**—Have thicker emulsion therefore they are faster and used in cardboard holders. These should always be manually processed. The screen films have more speed and contrast but less latitude (Range of exposure) than non-screen films.
3. **Mammography film**—These are single coated slow speed film, as they are being exposed at low Kvp and high mAs. These are flexible films loaded in a cassette having air gap on its front side which acts as a grid. This air gap eliminates or reduces the amount of scattered radiations before reaching the X-ray film. They are used to examine the mammary glands in case of carcinoma breast.

   There are three types of mammography film which are recognized:

   a. Single sided emulsion which is designated for use without intensifying screen coated with a green-emitting rare earth phosphor.

   b. Single sided emulsion designated for use with a single blue emitting intensifying screen, having fine grain characteristics.

   c. A duplitised emulsion containing more silver and having greater sensitivity to direct X-radiation.
4. **Dental film**

   Intra-oral and Panoramic. They may be necessary for certain specialized equipment associated with rotational tomography of the jaws, when the film must be bent to a shape correspondent to the right and left halves of the maxilla considered simultaneously.

   The flexible cassette is a simple envelop of plastic material, folded at one end and fastened with press buttons of conventional design. It is an uncomplicated and practical piece or equipment. These type of the cassette are easy to fix according to the structure of the part. They can be in good but not uniform contact with the object or the part. Small flexible cassettes are used for dental radiography. The knob on the front side should coincide with the crown of the teeth. The approximate sizes of these flexible cassettes are 3 cm × 4 cm, 5 cm × 7 cm used for the routine dental radiography and 30 cm × 12 cm (12" × 5") and 30 cm × 15 cm (12" × 6") are used in panromax radiography.

There is no intensifying screen present in these cassettes and are exposed directly to x-radiations. The film is wrapped in a black paper. On its back portion lead foil is installed to absorp the radiation to avoid back scatter radiation. The film all together is sealed in a plastic envelop.

5. **Duplicating film**—It is single emulsion film that is exposed to ultraviolet light through the existing radiography to produce a copy.
6. **Subtraction film**.
7. **Medical imaging film**—Single coated film and has got five layers:
   a. Polyester base.
   b. Substratum.
   c. Emulsion.
   d. Top coat (gelatin and hardener).
   e. Back layer is *antiholo.*

Different size of film available:

17" × 14"	10" × 8"
15" × 12"	6½" × 8½"
12" × 12"	15" × 6"
12" × 10"	11" × 14"
	14" × 14"

Digital Radiography

In this form of imaging system, digital X-ray sensors are used in place of old method of X-ray photographic film. Its main advantage is time efficiency as it does not require chemical processing and drying technique. It digitally transfer and enhance images. It reduces radiation quantity for producing an image of similar contrast as compared with the conventional radiography.

In place of X-ray film, it uses a digital image capture device which gives advantages of image preview and availability at a faster rate and skips the costly affair for the chemicals and time efficiently and improving of image quality of desired level.

Direct Digital Detectors most commonly used are Flat Panel Detectors (FPDs) classified in two main categories:

1. **Indirect FPDs:** The most commonly used material in this FPDs is Amorphous silicon. It is combined with a scintillator in the outer layer made from a type of rare earth phosphor like caesium iodide (CsI) or gadolinium oxysulfide (Gd_2O_2S), as these have the ability to convert X-rays to light photons. This is the reason that Amorphous silicon detector is considered as an indirect imaging device. The light is directed through Amorphous silicon photodiode layer and is converted to a digital output signal. This digital signal is then read out by thin film transistors (TFTs) or fiber-coupled CCDs.
2. **Direct FPDs:** The material most often chosen for Direct FPDs is Amorphous selenium and the electric charge produced following X-ray interaction is detected by an array of pixels each consisting of an electrode and a capacitor. This charge produced is stored in each capacitor until it is read-out by the electronic switching circuitry. The photoconductor requires a voltage of approx. 5,000 V to be applied, using a surface electrode, so that the charge produced can be attracted to the pixel electrodes. as they can directly convert X-ray photons into charge. The outer layer of the flat panel is a high-voltage bias electrode. X-ray photons create electron-hole pairs in Amorphous selenium. The potential of the bias voltage charge

affects the transition of these electrons and holes. The holes are replaced with electrons and the resultant charge pattern in the selenium layer is read out by a TFT array, active matrix array, electrometer probes or microplasma line addressing.

Dry films are composed of a 175 micron-thick Polyester base and coated with silver salts and a protective layer, making it resistant to scratches and moisture. The PET base (polyethylene terephthalate-PET) with rounded corners ensures that the film can be handled in the same way as regular X-ray films. The silver based imaging layer is heat-sensitive but not light-sensitive. It ensures low fog and high contrast. It is convenient, environmentally friendly and cost-effective.

No wet processing or darkroom, eliminating cleaning products, time-consuming adjustments and chemical disposal. Smooth workflow and improved productivity is ensured. The films of different formats need not to be continuously re-loaded again and again, which makes for a smoother workflow. It has blue base with a maximum optical density of less than 4 and can be loaded in the daylight (films are insensitive to light).

Cassette

In construction of a typical cassette, a steel or aluminium frame supports a tray shaped front which forms a shallow container for one intensifying screen and an X-ray film (Thickness of sheet is about 1.2 mm). The front of the cassette naturally must be trans-radiant. The front sheet should be plastic laminated for protection from scratches and ease of cleaning. The back of the cassette is metal heavier gauge of aluminium and usually is lined with lead in order to protect the film from radiation scattered backwards from a bucky tray or other surface.

- On the inside of the back of the cassette is fixed black felt or plastic foam pad, to which is attached back intensifying screen. The function of the pad is to provide uniform contact of the X-ray film with the intensifying screen.
- Size of the cassette are available in the corresponding size of films.

Intensifying Screen

An intensifying screen is a device that absorbs and converts the incident X-ray photons into visible light. This visible light interacts with the radiographic film, forming the latent image, the intensifying screen acts as an amplifier of the remnant radiation reaching the screen film cassette. Use of an intensifying screen results in considerably lower radiation dose and on other hand increase the radiographic contrast.

There are four layers:

1. **Protective**—This is transparent layer of the screen. It makes the screen resistant to abrasion and damage caused by handling.
2. **Phosphor**—The active layer emits light during stimulation by X-rays. The active substance of conventional phosphor is crystalline calcium tungstate. Rare earth are the other phosphor material in newer faster screens.
3. **Reflective layer**—Between the phosphor and the base is a reflective layer approximately 25 μm thick, made of a substance such as magnesium oxide or titanium dioxide.
4. **Base**—It is 1 mm thick and serves principally as a mechanical support or phosphor layer.

Screen Speed

A screen is said to be fast when a relatively small X-ray exposure produces a given output of light and causes certain degree of blackening of film.

$$IF = \frac{\text{Exposure without screens}}{\text{Exposure with screen}}$$

Conventional screens are available in 5 speeds:

• Ultra speed	200
• High speed	100
• Medium speed	50
• Detail speed	35
• Ultra detail	15

Fluorescent Screen: In fluoroscopy, the visible light emitted by screen is viewed directly by radiologist and give the corresponding X-ray pattern. The intensity of light emitted by the screen is very low and therefore difficult to see and the eyes are most sensitive to green part of spectrum. Therefore, fluorescent material used is Zinc Cadmium Sulphide.

Hanger
- Clip type
- Channel type

ACQUISITION OF RADIOGRAPH

a. *Production of a Latent Image:* The central process is breaking of bromine barrier is an invisible change brought about by a patterned emergent X-ray beam on the radiation sensitive emulsion of a film. It is essentially bringing about a chemical change.

b. *Development:* Development is the process during which the latent image is converted into a realistic, static and permanent radiographic image. This is brought about by the conversion of exposed silver halide particles to a tiny opaque black silver speck.

c. *Fixation:* Fixation is the dissolution-off of the unexposed crystals on the film. If this is not done, then the ambient radiation would slowly convert the remaining unaffected crystals also to exposed ones and the contrast would be lost (a process called as Fogging). The film is simultaneously hardened.

d. *Washing and Drying:* Removal of useless chemicals. These processes are very important from a storage point of view. This preserves the manifest image steps (b) and (c) which produce it.

DARK-ROOM CHEMISTRY

Developer—It is reasonably strong reducing agent which can donate electrons preferentially to the silver halide crystals with a broken bromine barrier (Exposed silver bromide crystal). The term preferentially has a special meaning as a developer can denote to unexposed crystals also and therefore cause fogging effect, if allowed to act unduly on a film (i.e., for increased time, temperature and concentration). It is composed of:

1. *Organic Reducing Agent*
   - Hydroquinone (Late acting) + Metol/Elon (Early and quick acting developer) for manual processing.
   - Hydroquinone + Phenidone for automatic processing.
   - Hydroquinone is actually responsible for density built up (over a faint gray image formed by Metol) and therefore the ultimate film contrast. Unduly long and short times will lead to a dense or faint images respectively.
2. *Preservative*—Sodium Sulphite (Na_2SO_3).
   - It prevents developer from being oxidized by air.
   - It prevents staining of film by decomposition products in developer.
3. *Accelerator*—Sodium carbonate Na_2CO_3/NaOH.

   It swells up the gelatin and making the diffusion in developer and out of bromine etc. easily.
4. *Restrainer*—KBr potassium bromide—It prevents fogging.

The process of manual development is strictly time and temperature dependent (5 minutes at 20°C temperature) and so-called as time-temperature development. Frequent inspection during development should be avoided, however can be used only in dire emergency as it leads to fogging. Below 16°C, Hydroquinone stops acting while above 24°C the emulsion is softened leading to chemical fog. The time can be decided accordingly by standard charts. A non-screen film needs longer time. Gelatin agitation should be done to remove bromine and other products that stop uniform development and hence streaking of film.

Replenisher

A solution slightly different from developer which is added periodically. It maintains the strength by chemically acting with hydroquinone and metol and reduce the volume by carrying away some developer with it (75 ml developer is required for the development of one film of 17 × 14" size film).

Replenisher = Developer – Potassium bromide.

It differs from developer as:

1. It has no bromide (restrainer).
2. It has excess of hydroquinone, metol and alkali.

A developer can be used for 2-3 months with adequate addition of replenisher. Maximum re-plenishment that can be done upto volume of 4 times of developer.

Rinsing—Rinsing of the film after development can be done by running water or 1% acetic acid (CH_3COOH) solution. This is done to remove the developer from the film so that the acid in fixer is not degraded and the fixer can act uniformly.

Fixer—An acidic solution that removes the undeveloped silver halides, hardens the film and preserved the image. It is composed of:

1. *Fixer agent:*
   - Hypo (Sodium Thiosulphate)—Powder form.
   - Ammonium Thiosulfate–liquid.
   - Actually removes the under developed silver halide leading to the increase in contrast.
2. *Preservative*—Na_2SO_3.
3. *Hardener*—Chrome alum or potassium for hardening (or tanning) the gelatin.

4. **Acid**—Sulfuric acid/acetic acid.
   - It neutralizes the still present alkaline or developer.
   - It enables action of fixing agent and hardener.

Fixation time dependent upon fixer age and number of films fixed and is equal to cleaning time (1-4 minutes) + hardening time (2-8 minutes). This is more for a non-screen film. If fixer takes more time (> 10 minutes), remove it.

Agitation should be done to have a uniform action and light should not be allowed before 1 minute of fixation.

Prolonged fixation leads to firm adherence of hypo to film leading to an ultimate brownish gray tan (because of silver sulphide formation) or film is bleached. Temperature duration and image is same as that for developer. In actual the fixer should be in excess of developer and first forms a complex molecule with unexposed silver halide and removes it. This should also be replenished by new fixer solution.

Washing—For 20 minutes at 20°C in running water (40 minutes for non-screen film) rate of 6 times the tank volume per minute. Can be hastened by using a fixer neutralizer before washing.

FILM FOGS

a. **Due to exposure to light**
   - Dark-room is not light proof.
   - Safe light contains too large a bulb.
   - Safe light housing or filter is cracked.
   - Prolonged exposure of film to safe light.
   - Safe light series incorrect.

b. **Exposure to X-rays or other radioactive elements**—Films should be shielded from radioactive material by adequate thickness of lead and/or distance.

c. Chemical fog

- Over development.
- Development at high temperature.
- Oxidized deteriorated developer.
- Prolonged and repeated inspection of film during development.
- Contamination from old tank specially a porus type.

d. Age fog

- Mottled or uniformly foggy film due to use of expiry date film or storage under improper temperature or humidity etc.

DARK-ROOM ARTEFACTS

Stains

These are discolorations, that may appear on a film at different intervals after processing. These can be avoided by the use of fresh solution and using correct processing techniques.

- **Brown stains**—due to oxidized developer.
- **Variegated color pattern**—due to inadequate rinsing.
- **Grayish yellow or brown stains**—due to excessive fixation or use of exhausted fixer.
- **Grayish white scum**—due to incomplete washing.

Marks and Defects

a. **Crinkle (kink) marks**—Curved black lines about 1 cm long which results from the bending of the film acutely over the edge of finger.

b. **Static marks**—Tree like branching black marks on the film caused by static electricity, i.e., friction between the two films, a film and screen, a film and its cover.

c. **Water marks**—Droplets of water on film surface that may leave round spots of various size before exposing of the film or even after exposure, but before processing.

d. **Cassette marks**—Dust particle, fragments of paper, hair, defects on the screen all may leave a white spot of corresponding size on the film.

e. **Reticulation marks**—These are the networks of fine grooves on the film surface caused by marked difference in temperature of developing solutions.

f. **Streaking**—is due to:
   - Failure to agitate the film in developer.
   - Failure to rinse the film adequately.
   - Failure to agitate the film when first immersed in the fixer.
   - Failure to stir the solution thoroughly after preparation and replacement.

g. **Frilling**—Loosening of the gelatin from the base round the edge due to exhausted fixer, warm fixer, increased room temperature.

h. **Stripling**—Whole of the gelatin coating becoming detached.

MAXIMUM PERMISSIBLE DOSE (MPD)

Maximum permissible dose is defined as the maximum dose of ionizing radiation which an individual may receive without suffering appreciable bodily injury during his life time.

The accumulated occupational MPD from X, Gamma or Beta radiation to the whole body and to certain radiosensitive organs like gonads, blood forming organs, lens of eye and trunk shall not exceed

$$MPD = 5\ (N - 18)\ \text{rads}$$

Where N is the age in years and is more than 18. For example, at the age of 32 years MPD is 5 (32 – 18) = 70 rads. Average annual MPD is 5 rads, weekly 0.1 rad or 100 millirads. An accumulated dose of 3 rads is allowed in **"any 13 weeks period"**. The hand and feet may receive as much as 75 rads per year; but not more than 25 rads in **"any 13 weeks period"**. The above requirements apply only to radiation workers. The MPD for general population is 1/10 of the above limits. The radiation exposure of X-ray personnel for their own diagnosis and therapy is not included in calculating the MPD.

2

Radiographic Positioning

A few **common terminologies** which are used; commonly in practice, should be familiar to every radiology technician.

Anatomical Terminology

Anterior aspect is that seen when viewing the patient from the front. Posterior aspect is that when viewing the patient from the back. Lateral aspect refers to the view of the patient from the side; thus we have a lateral aspect of the head (side of the head) or the trunk. Similarly, we have the outer surface as lateral aspect of the limb while the inner side of the limb is its medial aspect.

Planes of the Body

The three planes described are mutually at right angles to each other, the median sagittal plane is a plane which divides the body into right and left halves.

A coronal plane divides the body into an anterior part and posterior part. A transverse plane divides the body into a superior part and an inferior part.

Positioning Terminology

This describes how the patient is positioned for the projection to be taken. The patient may be decubitus (Lying down), erect (sitting or standing) or semi-recumbent.

If decubitus, the patient may be:

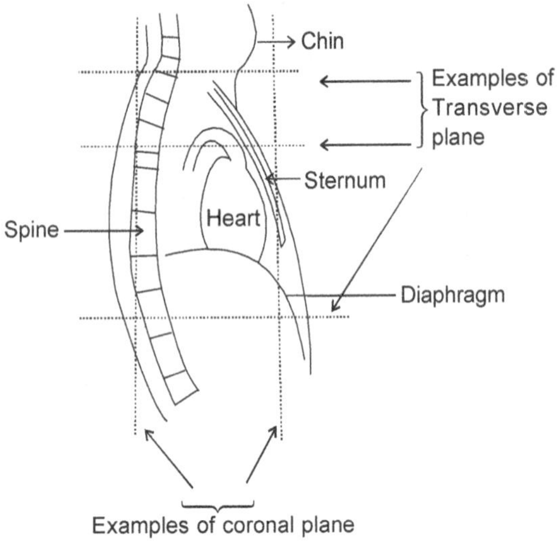

Fig. 2.1: Sagittal section

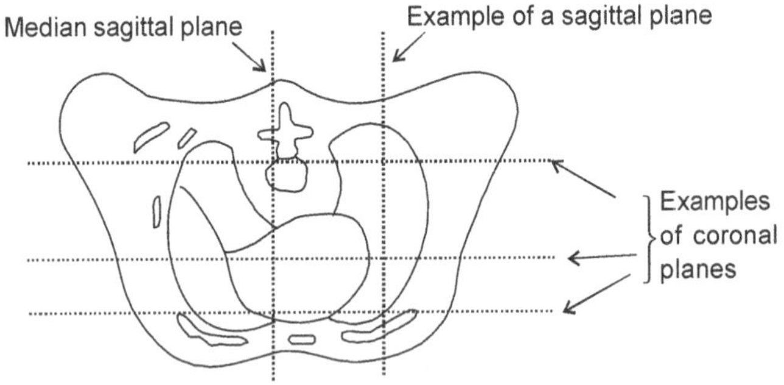

Fig. 2.2: Transverse section

1. Supine (dorsal decubitus)—Lying on back.
2. Prone (ventral decubitus)—Lying face down.
3. Lateral decubitus—Lying on the side. Right lateral decubitus—Lying on the right side. Left lateral decubitus—Lying on the left side.

In the erect position, the patient may be standing or sitting:

1. With the posterior aspect against the film.
2. With the anterior aspect against the film.
3. With the right or left side against the film.

Projection Terminology

A projection is described by the direction of the central ray relative to aspects and planes of the body.

Anteroposterior (AP)

The central ray is incident on the anterior aspect; passes along a transverse plane and along or parallel to the median sagittal plane and emerges from the posterior aspect.

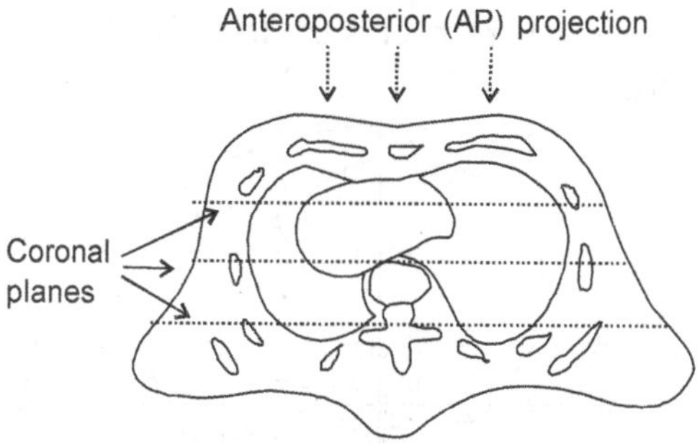

Fig. 2.3

Posteroanterior (PA)

The central ray is incident on the posterior aspect; passes along a transverse plane and along or parallel to the median sagittal plane and emerges from the anterior aspect.

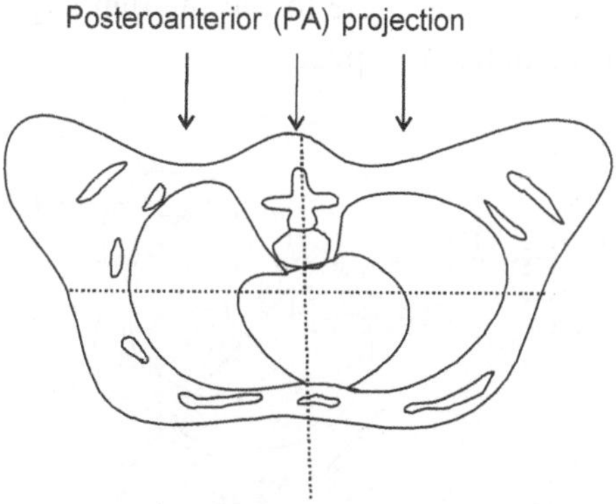

Fig. 2.4

Lateral

The central ray passes from one side of the body to the other along a coronal and transverse plane. The projection is called a right lateral if the central ray passes from left side to right side and a left lateral if the central ray passes from right side to left side.

In the case of a limb, the central ray is either incident on the lateral aspect and emerges from the medial aspect (lateromedial), or is incident on the medial aspect and emerges from the lateral aspect of the limb (mediolateral). The terms 'lateromedial' and mediolateral are used where necessary to differentiate between the two projections.

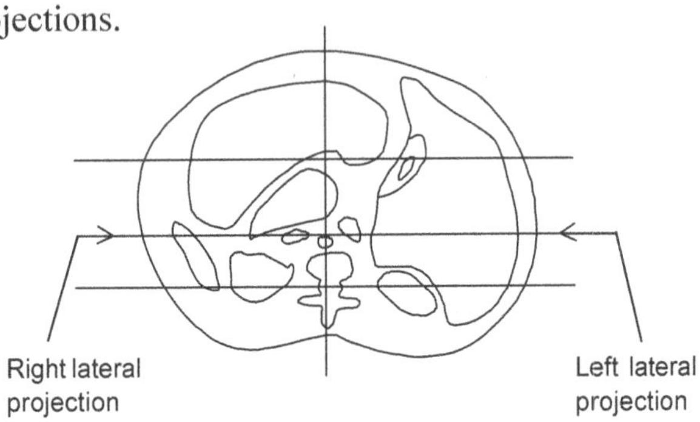

Fig. 2.5

Anterior Oblique

The central ray enters the posterior aspect, passes along a transverse plane at some angle to the median sagittal plane and emerges from the anterior aspect.

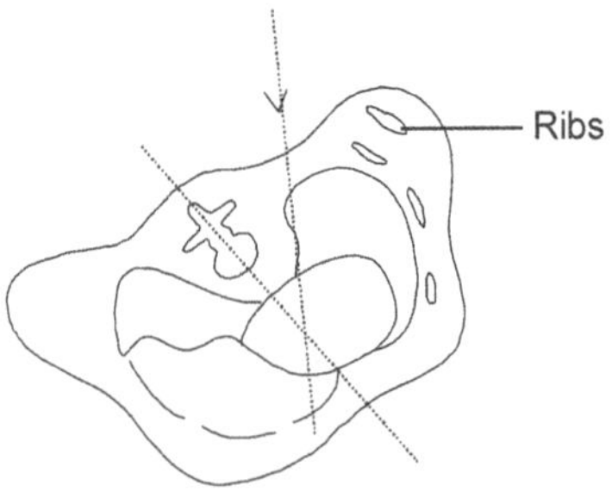

Fig. 2.6a: Right anterior oblique

Posterior Oblique

The central ray enters the anterior aspect, passes along a transverse plane at some angle to the median sagittal plane and emerges from the posterior aspect.

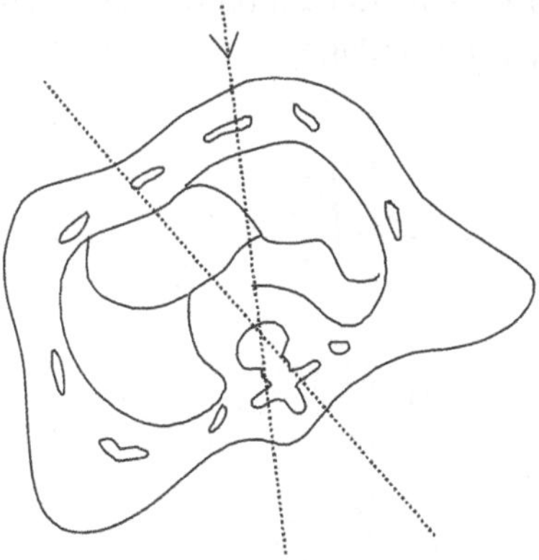

Fig. 2.6b: Left posterior oblique

When the patient prone and the median sagittal plane at right angles to the film; right and left anterior oblique projections are obtained by angling the central ray to the median sagittal plane.

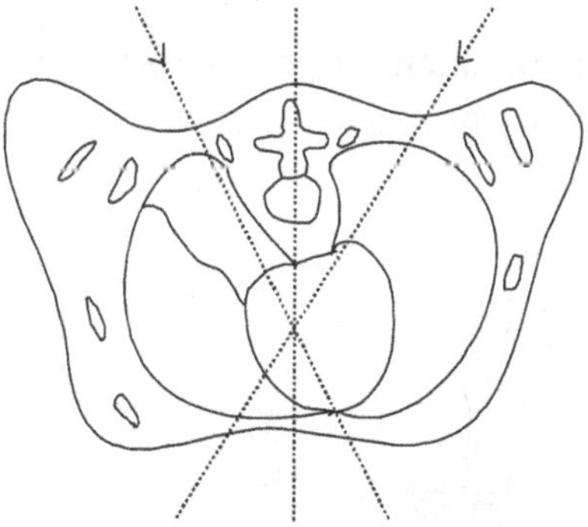

Fig. 2.7: Right or left anterior oblique

Oblique

The central ray passes through the body along a transverse plane at some angle between the median sagittal and coronal planes. For this projection the patient is usually positioned with the median sagittal plane at some angle between 0 and 90 degrees to the film and the central ray is at right angles to the films. The patient is positioned with the median sagittal plane at right angles to or parallel to the film and the projection is obtained directing the central ray at some angle to the median sagittal plane.

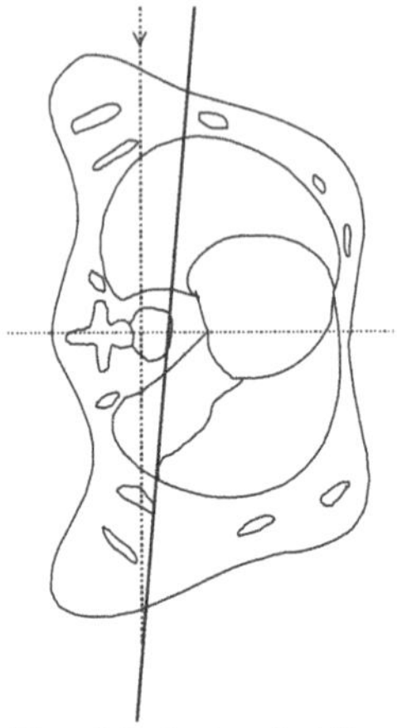

Fig. 2.8: Lateral oblique

Lateral Oblique

The central ray enters on lateral aspect, passes along transverse plane at an angle to the coronal plane and emerges from the opposite lateral aspect.

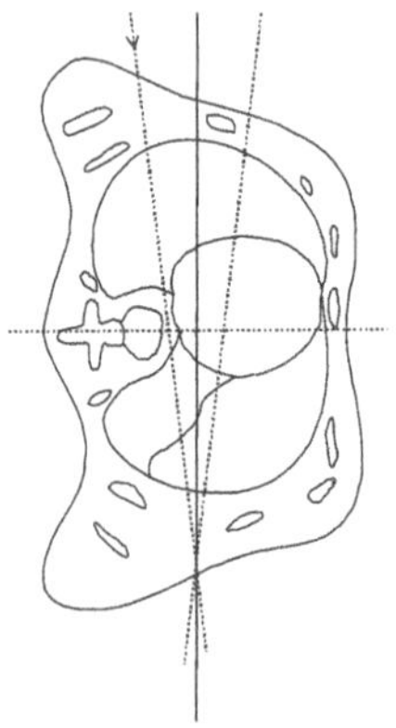

Fig. 2.9: Coronal plane

With the coronal plane at right angles to the film, lateral oblique projections are obtained by angling the central ray to the coronal plane.

To describe how a radiographic projection is obtained, it is necessary to give:

1. The position of the patient related to the film.
2. The direction and centering of the X-ray beam. The direction and centering of the X-ray beam is given by reference to an imaginary central ray of the X-ray beam which can be assessed with the help of the collimated light beam.

   In brief the terms mentioned can be understood as:

   (a) *Anterior*: Towards the front side of the body.

   (b) *Posterior*: Towards the back side of the body.

   (c) *Superior*: Towards the head side.

   (d) *Inferior*: Towards the feet.

   (e) *Medial*: Towards the median plane of the body.

   (f) *Lateral*: Away from the median plane of the body.

   (g) *Ventral*: Towards the belly, like anterior part of the body.

   (h) *Dorsal*: Towards the spine or like posterior side of the body.

   (i) *Cranial*: Towards the head or like superior part of the body.

   (j) *Caudal*: Towards the tail of the body.

   The other commonly used terms includes:

   (a) *Proximal*: Nearer or closer to the trunk.

   (b) *Distal*: Away or at distant from the trunk.

   (c) *Radial*: It is the outer border of the upper limb when in true anatomical position.

   (d) *Ulnar*: It is the inner border of the upper limb, when in true anatomical position.

   (e) *Flexor*: It is the anterior surface in the upper limb and posterior surface of the lower limb.

   (f) *Extensor*: It is the posterior surface in the upper limb and anterior surface of the lower limb.

   (g) *Palmar*: Towards the palms of the hand.

(h) *Plantar*: Towards the sole of the foot.

(i) *Interior*: Inner.

(j) *Exterior*: Outer.

(k) *Superficial*: Towards the surface of the body.

(l) *Deep*: Towards the inner layers of the body.

(m) *Ipsilateral*: The same side.

(n) *Contralateral*: The opposite side.

The body movements are described by the following terms:

(a) *Adduction*: Movement towards the central axis or towards the body.

(b) *Abduction*: Movement away from the body or away from central axis.

(c) *Flexion*: It is the term to reduce the angulations of the joint.

(d) *Extension*: Used to increase the angulations of the joint.

(e) *Medial Rotation*: Inward rotation.

(f) *Lateral Rotation*: Outward rotation.

(g) *Pronation*: Rotation of the forearm so that the palm of the hand is turned backward.

(h) *Supination*: Rotation of the forearm so that the palm of the hand is turned forward.

The other common terms used in various positioning of the patient in radiography are as under:

(a) *Axial*: Angulation of the X-ray beam in the direction of the body axis.

(b) *Dorsi-Plantar*: In case of the foot the X-rays are directed from top of the foot towards the back or lower side of the foot. In *planti-dorsal* the X-rays are directed from the lower side of the foot (planter) to the top of the foot.

(c) *Decubitus*: The patient lies on the lateral side of his body to see the fluid level in the pleural cavity and the cassette is placed vertically in front or behind the patient.

To get the complete information of the part to be radiograph, it is usually done by two or more views.

HEAD AND NECK

To obtain different skiagram of skull, some of the basic lines are to be considered:

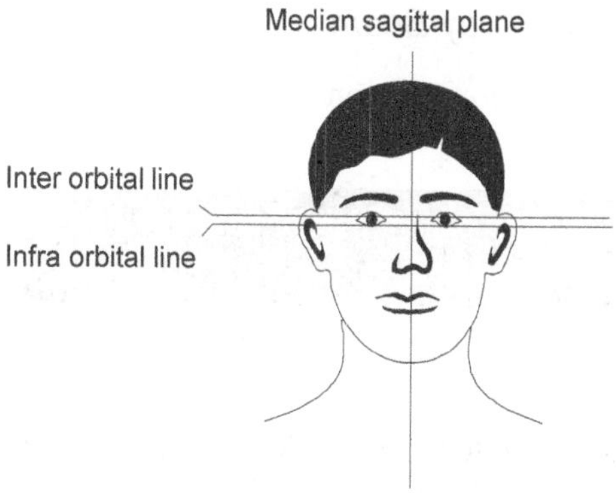

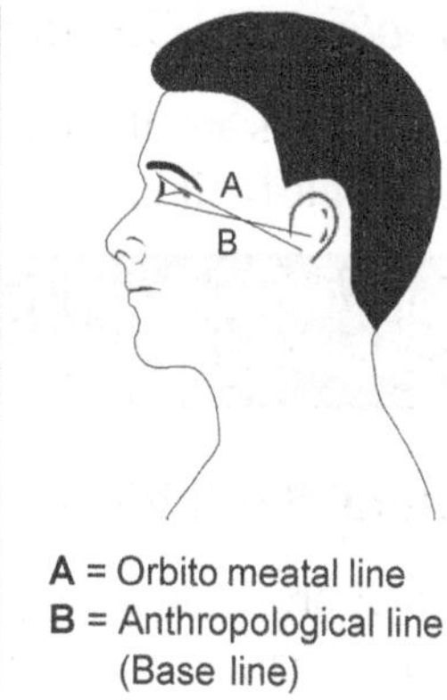

Posteroanterior View of Skull

(Occipitofrontal View)

Patient lies prone on the table with chin touching the X-ray table with canthomeatal line perpendicular to table top.

Central ray: 2.5 cm above external occipital protuberance with straight X-ray tube.

Distance 90 cm KvP 70 mAs 60

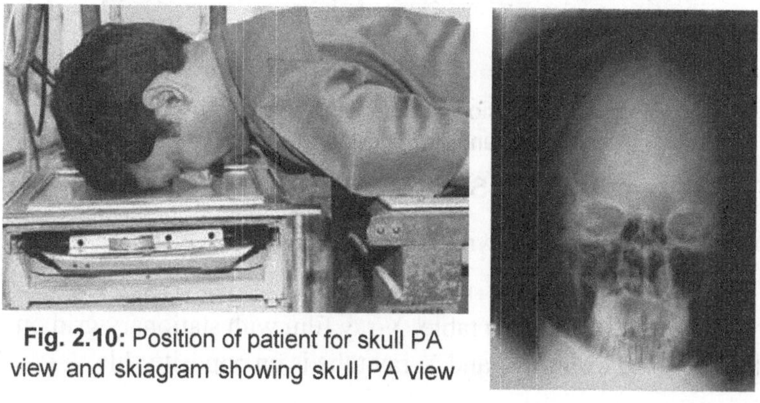

Fig. 2.10: Position of patient for skull PA view and skiagram showing skull PA view

Anteroposterior or Fronto-occipital View of Skull

Patient lies supine on table with chin slightly tilted downward toward the chest so as to make canthomeatal line perpendicular to the film.

Direction and Centring of the X-ray Beam

Central rays are aligned 2 inches above nasion or bridge of nose at right angle to film.

Note: Generally employed when the patient cannot lie prone either because of injury or comatosed/paralysed.

Lateral Skull View

Patient prone on table. Head is rotated to the side to be examined with median sagittal plane is parallel with table and inter pupillary line is at right angles to the film. Raise the shoulder of the side towards which the head is rotated and supported with sandbag.

Central ray: 1" in front of and ½" above external auditory meatus (Fig. 2.11).

Distance 90 cm KvP 70 mAs 40-50

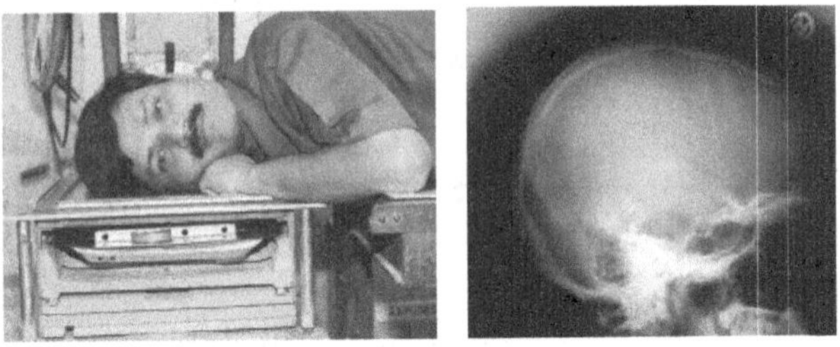

Fig. 2.11: Position of patient for lateral view skull and skiagram showing lateral view skull

Translateral View of Skull

Also known as cone-down view for sella turcica or supine lateral view of skull.

Patient lies supine on table. X-ray film with stationary grid on the side to be examined and X-ray tube is on opposite side.

Direction and centring of the X-ray beam: Central rays 1" in front of external auditory meatus. Exposure factor same as in lateral view.

Towne's View (Half-axial View) (AP View 30° Tube Tilt): Patient lies supine on the table with chin is made down to touch the chest so that canthomeatal line is made right angle to film.

Direction and centring of the X-ray beam: Central rays are aligned at a point 5 cm above glabella or bridge of nose with X-ray tube lilted 30° towards caudally. Patient is asked to hold the breath during exposure.

Distance 90 cm KvP 86 mAs 80

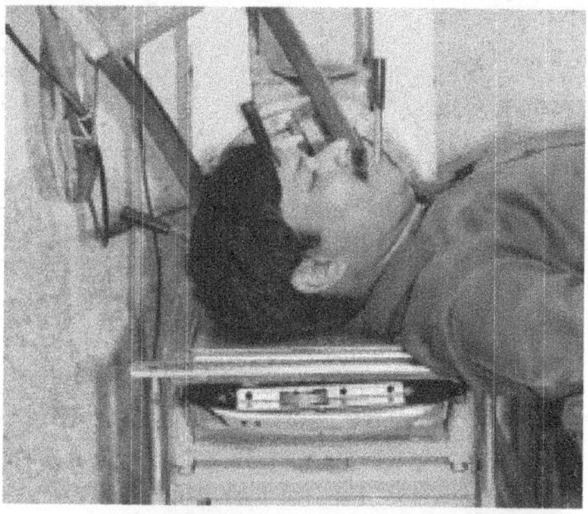

Fig. 2.12a: Patient's position for Towne's view

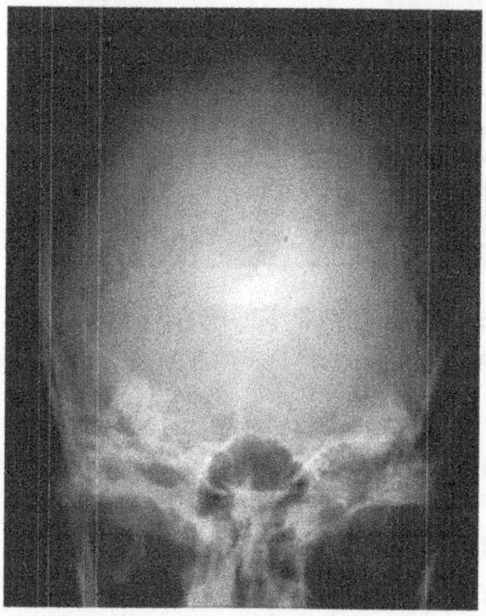

Fig. 2.12b: Skiagram showing skull in Towne's view

Reverse Towne's View

Patient lies prone, with orbitomeatal is perpendicular and chin touching the chest.

Direction and centring of the X-ray beam: Central rays passes 30° caudal tilt through bridge of nose.

Distance 90 cm KvP 86 mAs 80

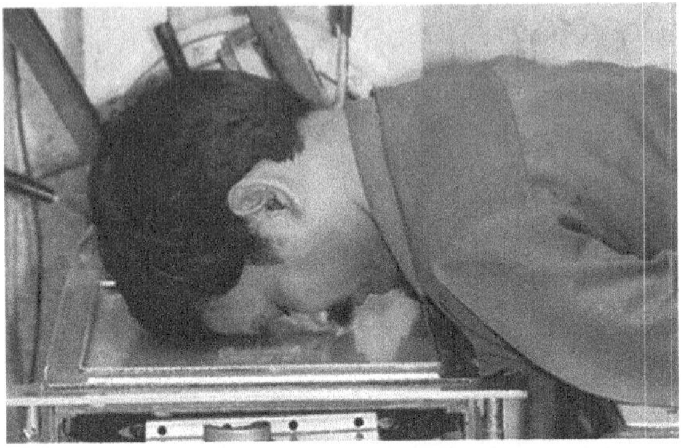

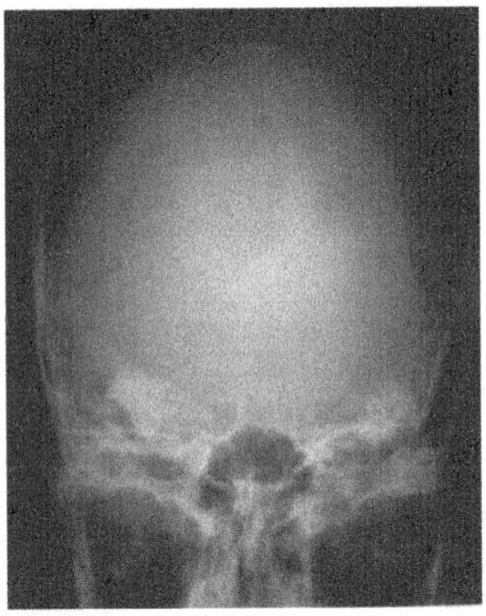

Fig. 2.13: Patient's position for reverse Towne's view and skiagram to show Towne's reverse view

Submentovertical View/Basal View/Base of Skull

Patient lies supine on table with neck is kept hyperextended so that canthomeatal line becomes parallel to the table top. To achieve this position a pillow or sandbag is kept under the shoulder.

Direction and Centring of the X-ray Beam: Central ray is aligned to pass at midpoint of the line joining the two angles of the mandible at right angle to the film.

Distance 90 cm KvP 86 mAs 100

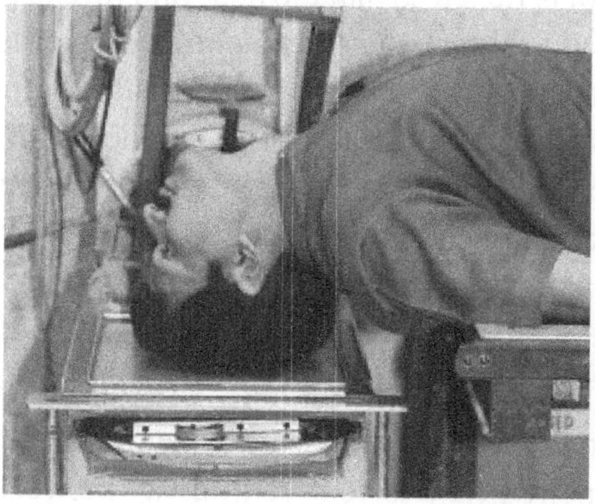
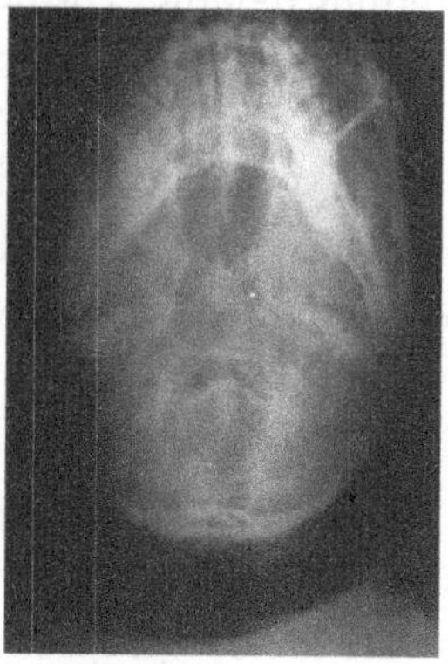

Fig. 2.14: Position of patient for basal view and skiagram for basal view or base of skull

Lateral Mastoid View (Schuller's View): Patient is prone (erect) with the head in true lateral position with median sagittal plane parallel to the film and interorbital line perpendicular to the film.

Direction and Centring of the X-ray Beam: Central ray: 2" above external auditory meatus, with tube angled 35° towards the feet.

Distance 90 cm KvP 76 mAs 60

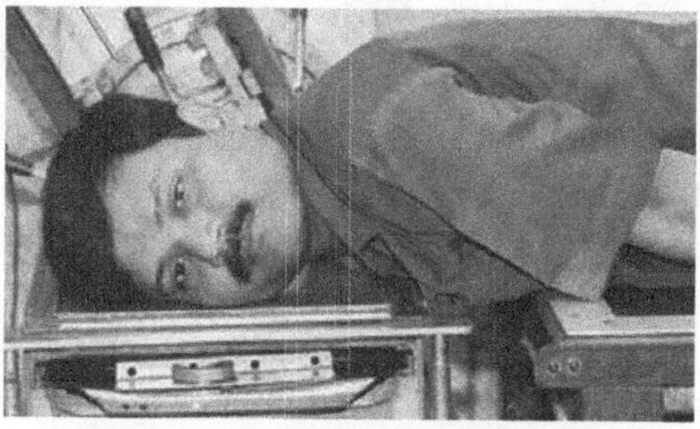
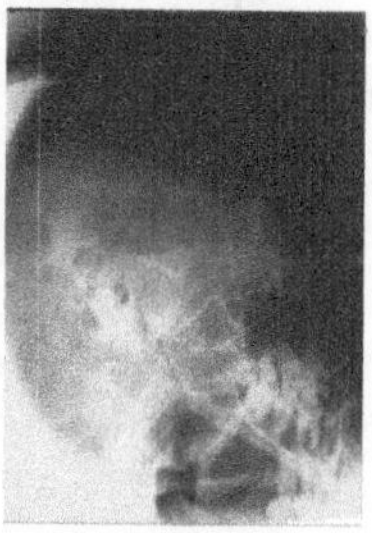

Fig. 2.15: Position of patient for lateral mastoid view and skiagram of lateral mastoid view

Stenver's View

Both Sides are Examined for Comparison: Patient is prone facing a film in bucky. The patient is adjusted in position so that the middle of supraorbital margin on the side being examined is centred to midline of table. The neck is flexed so that the nose and forehead are in contact with table and orbitomeatal line is perpendicular to table. The external auditory meatuses should be equidistant from the table so that the median sagittal plane is at right angles to the table. The neck is now extended slightly so that orbitomeatal line is at an angle of 5° to vertical and head is then rotated through 45° towards the side being examined to bring the superior border of petrous temporal bone parallel to the film.

Direction and Centring of the X-ray Beam: Central ray is angled 12° cephalad, i.e., at an angle of 7° to orbitomeatal plane, to separate the occiput from petrous and is centred midway between occipital protuberance and external auditory meatus. The beam should be collimated.

Distance 90 cm KvP 80 mAs 80

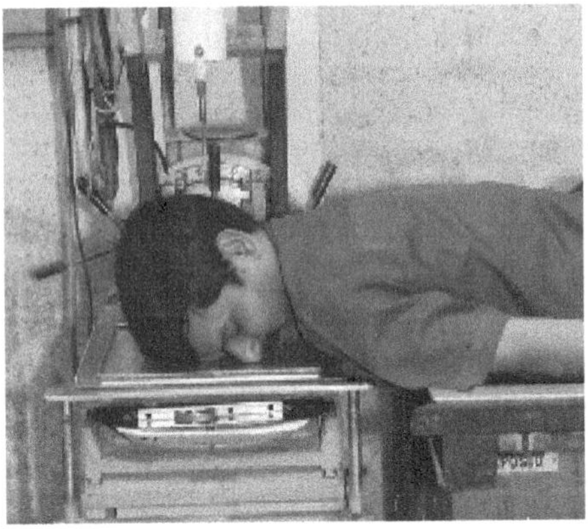

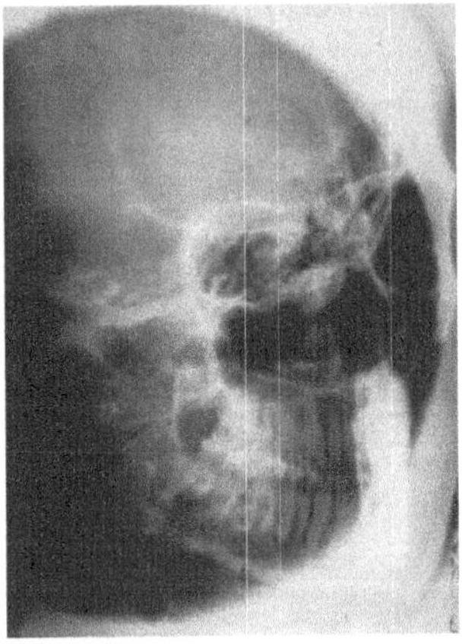

Fig. 2.16: Position of patient in Stenver's view and skiagram showing Stenver's view

Optic Foramina View: Patient lies prone on the table. Place orbit of the side under examination directly over the film resting the forehead, cheek and nose on the table. Head is adjusted so that median sagittal plane and canthomeatal line make an angle of 35° with perpendicular plane.

Direction and Centring of the X-ray Beam: Central rays through orbit nearer the film, to pass through lower and outer quadrant of the orbit. Both sides are examined for comparison.

Both optic foramina should be examined to compare the diameter of optic foramen.

Distance 90 cm KvP 80 mAs 60

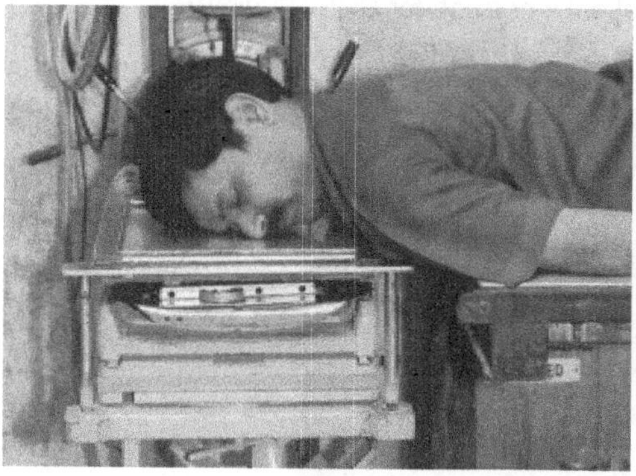

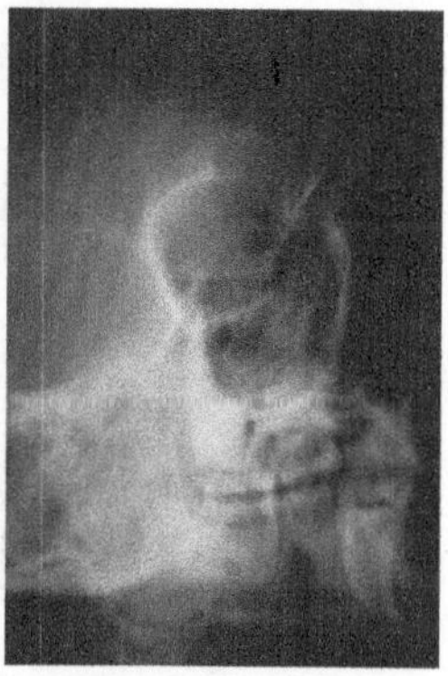

Fig. 2.17: Position of patient for right optic foramina and skiagram showing optic foramina of right side

Paranasal Sinuses (PNS) PA View

Patient lies prone on the table with flexed neck in such a way that canthomeatal line is 45° to the table top.

Direction and Centring of the X-ray Beam: Central ray are aligned over top of vertex.

Distance 90 cm KvP 80 mAs 80

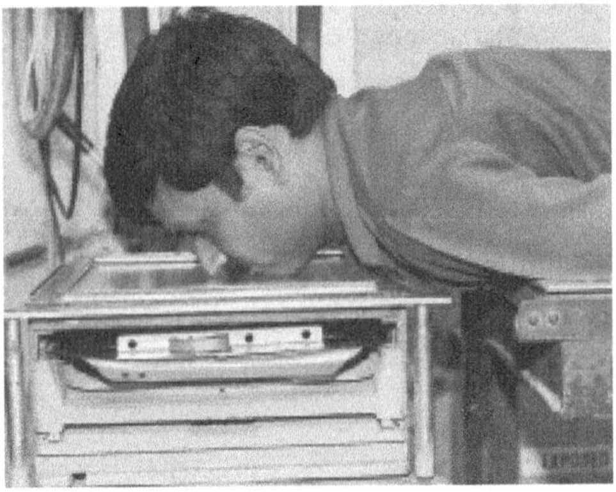

Fig. 2.18a: Patient's position for PNS PA view

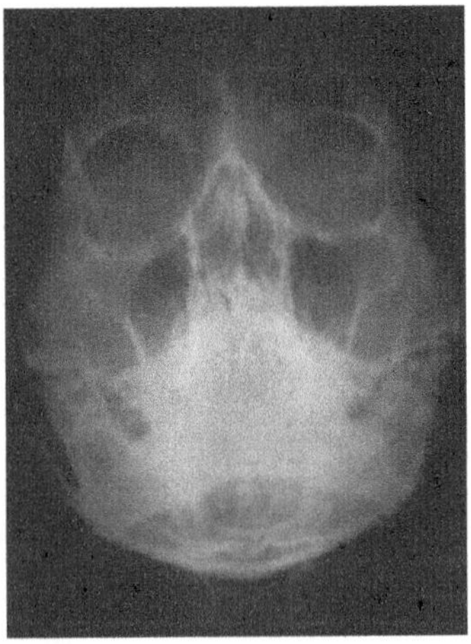

Fig. 2.18b: Skiagram showing paranasal sinuses (PNS) PA view

PNS 20° View

Patient lies prone on the table with same position as in standard PNS PA view.

Direction and Centring of the X-ray Beam: Central rays are aligned 20° caudally over top of vertex.

Distance 90 cm KvP 86 mAs 80

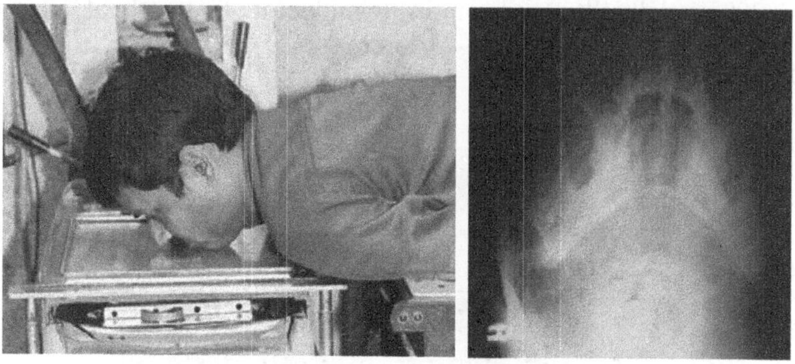

Fig. 2.19: Position of patient for PNS 20° or 30° and skiagram showing PNS 30° orbit view

Lateral View of PNS: Patient lies prone on table with head rotated to the side to be examined so that canthomeatal line becomes parallel to film.

Direction and Centring of the X-ray Beam: Central rays are aligned 2.5 cm behind outer canthus of eye at right angles to film.

Distance 90 cm KvP 72 mAs 50

Right and Left Oblique View (For Posterior Ethmoidal Sinuses): The head is placed with nose, forehead and cheek resting on table with canthomeatal line at right angle to the film. Rotate the head 40° to side to be examined. Raise the chin so that the canthomeatal line becomes at an angle of 30° to the film.

Direction and Centring of the X-ray Beam: Central rays over orbit nearer to the film (2.5 inch above and behind the external auditory meatus of the side away from film) at right angle to film.

Distance 90 cm KvP 80 mAs 60

PA 20° Orbit/20° Occipitofrontal/Inclined Postero-anterior/Caldwell View: Patient lies prone on table with head in true PA position having midline plane and canthomeatal line are perpendicular to the film.

Direction and Centring of the X-ray Beam: Central rays are 20° caudally tilted and pointing to midpoint of interorbital line.

Distance 90 cm KvP 80 mAs 80

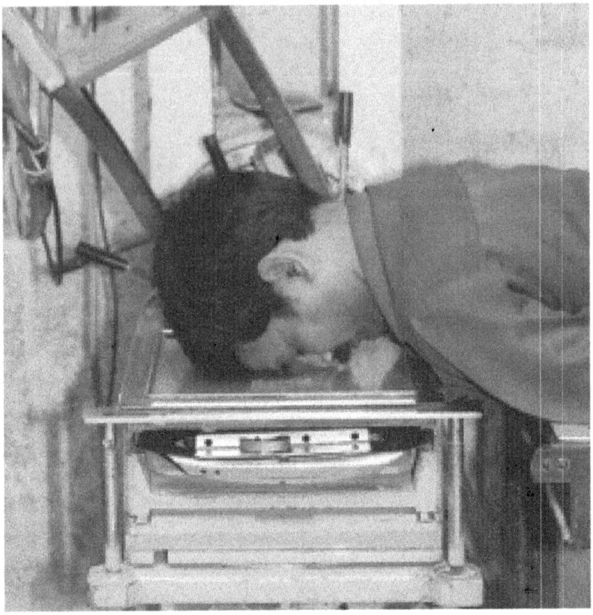

Fig. 2.20a: Position of patient for skull PA 20° orbital view

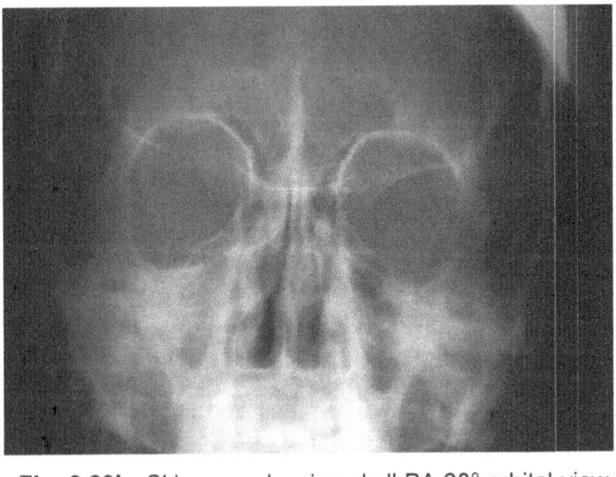

Fig. 2.20b: Skiagram showing skull PA 20° orbital view

Nasal Bone View: Patient lies prone on table with head rotated to right or left side so that median sagittal plane is parallel with the table and interorbital line is at right angle to film. Shoulder is to be raised and supported on sand bag. Care should be taken to see that the film is parallel with line of nasal septum, nose being in the centre of the film.

Direction and Centring of X-ray Beam: Central rays are over the root of nose and at right angles to film.

Distance 90 cm KvP 45 mAs 8-10

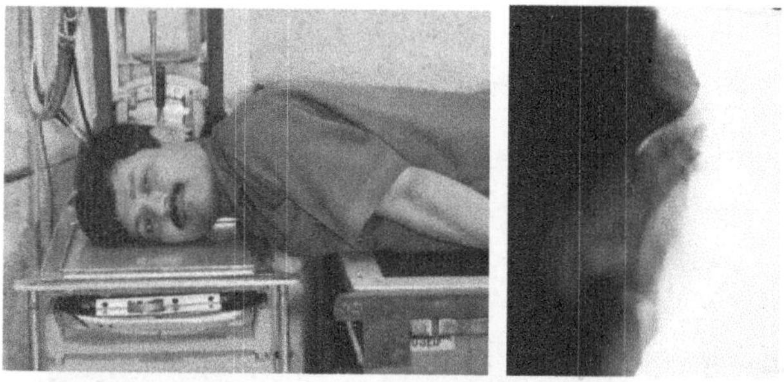

Fig. 2.21: Position of patient for nasal bone view

Posteroanterior View of Mandible: Patient lies prone on table. Canthomeatal line is at right angle to film and interpupillary line parallel with film. Care should be taken to see that both ear lobules are at equidistance with film.

Direction and Centring of X-ray Beam: Central ray to be aligned in midline, between the angle of mandible and passing through lips, perpendicular to the film.

Distance 90 cm KvP 70 mAs 60

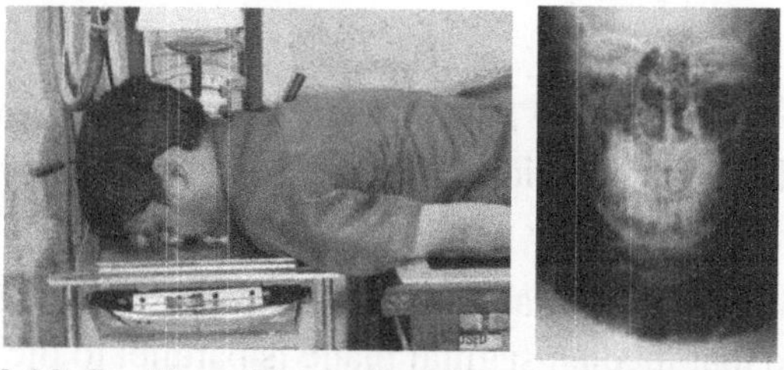

Fig. 2.22: Position of the patient for mandible AP view and skiagram of the same

Mandible Lateral Oblique View: Patient is supine on table. The head is rotated right or left depending upon which lateral oblique is required. Rotation is kept to median line is parallel with table. Interorbital line is perpendicular to film. Raise the shoulder of the side toward which the head has been rotated and support with sandbag.

Direction and Centring of X-ray Beam: Central ray: 2" below the angle of mandible farthest from the film of an angle of 30° cranially.

Distance 90 cm KvP 70 mAs 40

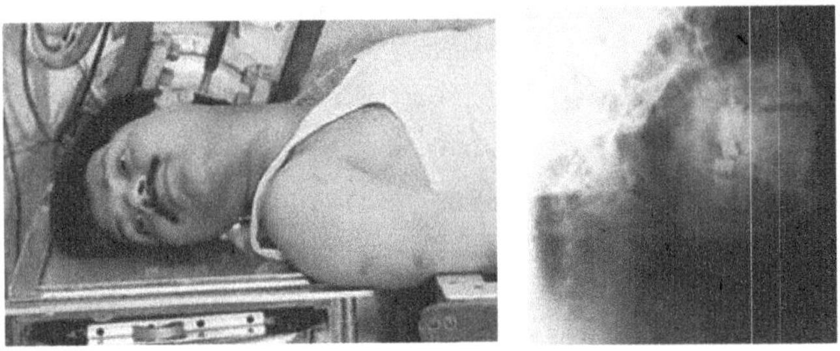

Fig. 2.23: Position of the patient for lateral oblique view of mandible and skiagram showing mandible in lateral oblique view

Symphysis Mentic View: Patient lies supine on table, an occlusal film is placed in the mouth as far back as possible and the mouth is gently closed with the film in between the teeth. Head is thrown back with neck in hyperextension and shoulders are raised from the table.

Direction and Centring of X-ray Beam: Central rays are aligned about 1" below the chin.

Distance 90 cm KvP 70 mAs 60

Temporomandibular Joint (TMJ) View: Always process it for both sides and each side to be examined in open mouth and closed mouth view.

Patient lies prone on table with head rotated to the side to be examined so that median sagittal plane is parallel to the table top. Interorbital line should be perpendicular to table, i.e., head should be in true lateral position.

Direction and Centring of X-ray Beam: Central rays are aligned over the TMJ nearest to film 2" above the external auditory meatus, away from the film at an angle of 20° towards the feet.

Distance 90 cm KvP 76 mAs 50

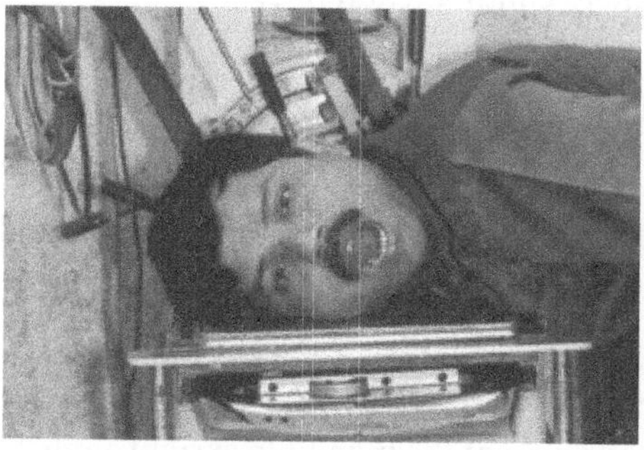
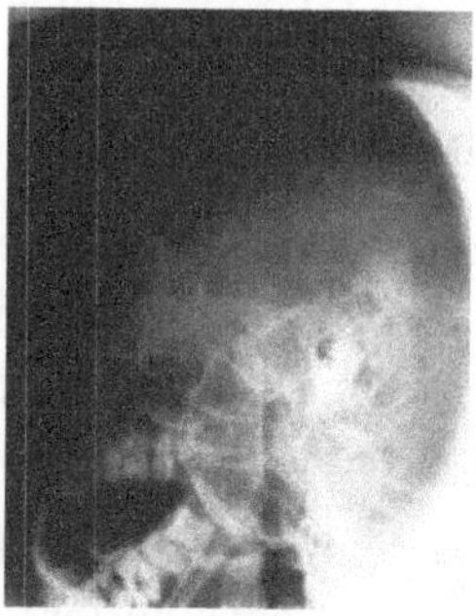

Fig. 2.24: Position of patient of right TMJ mouth open view and skiagram showing the same

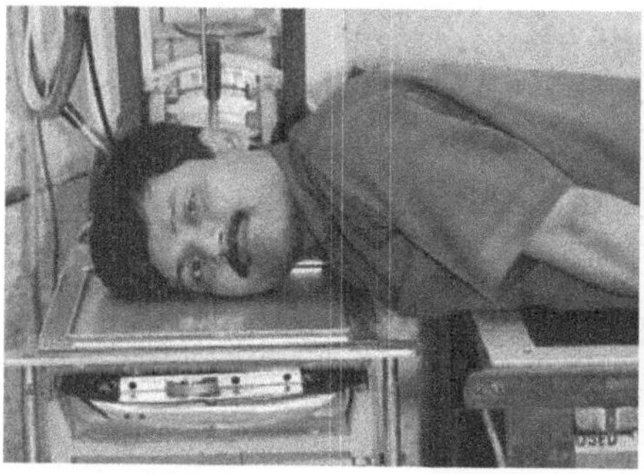
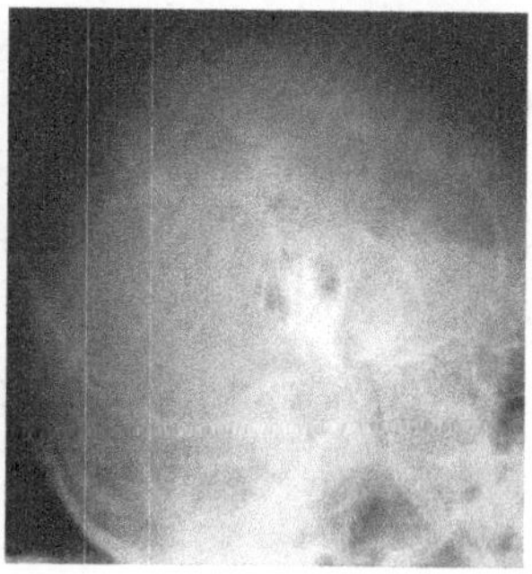

Fig. 2.25: Position of patient of right TMJ closed mouth view and skiagram showing the same

Anteroposterior View with 30° Tube Tilt for Zygomatic Process: Patient lies supine on table with chin put down so that canthomeatal line is right angle to film.

Direction and Centring of X-ray Beam: Central rays aligned to pass through glabella or bridge of nose at an angle of 30° toward feet.

Distance 90 cm KvP 80 mAs 60

Verticomental View: Patient sitting on table having chin resting on film. Then tilt the head backwards as much as possible so that canthomeatal line and interpupillary lines become parallel with film.

Direction and Centring of X-ray Beam: Central rays aligned through vertex at right angle to canthomeatal line.

Submandibular Gland

Lateral View: Patient lies prone on the X-ray table. Head is rotated to side in question with median sagittal plane is parallel to table and interorbital line perpendicular to the film. Raised shoulder should be supported with sandbag.

Direction and Centring of X-ray Beam: Central rays are aligned 2.5 cm anterior to the angle of the mandible at right angle to the film.

Distance 90 cm KvP 70 mAs 50

Inferosuperior (Occlusal) View: Patient lies supine on the table with neck and shoulder supported by sandbags and head thrown back as far as possible. An occlusal film is placed between the teeth as far back as possible and also covering greater part of the side under examination.

Direction and Centring of X-ray Beam: Central rays passes under the chin about 2.5 cm behind the point of chin at right angles to the film.

Sublingual Gland

Inferosuperior View: The patient lies supine on the table with neck and shoulders supported by sandbag and head thrown back as far as possible. An occlusal film is placed inside the mouth between the teeth, for enough back to get the 2nd molar tooth on the film.

Direction and Centring of X-ray Beam: Central rays passes under the chin about 2.5 cm back from the point of chin at right angles to the film.

Distance 90 cm KvP 70 mAs 50

SPINE OR VERTEBRAL COLUMN

Cervical Spine

Anteroposterior (Mouth Open) View (For C_1-C_2): Patient supine on table or erect facing the tube with median sagittal plane perpendicular to the film. The chin is raised slightly until canthomeatal line is tilted 10° from perpendicular.

Direction and Centring of X-ray Beam: Central rays are aligned through a widely open mouth at right angles to the film midway between the jaws.

Distance 90 cm KvP 76 mAs 40

Grid Yes

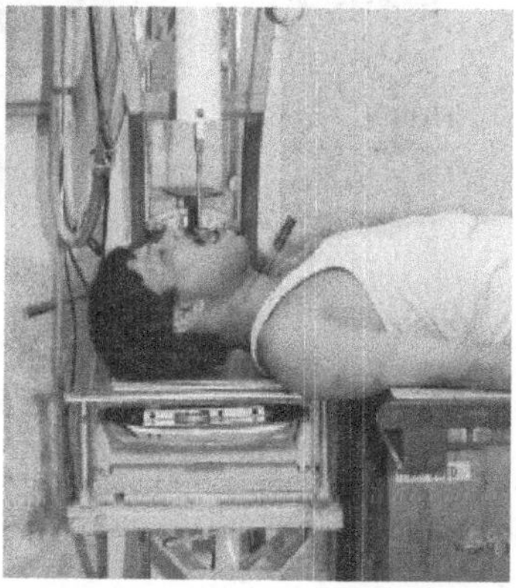
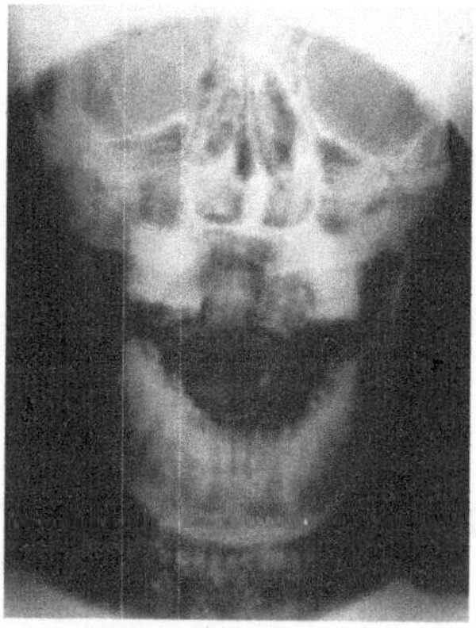

Fig. 2.26: Position of patient for C_1 and C_2 vertebrae in AP view and skiagram for mouth open view for C_1 and C_2

Anteroposterior View (C_3-C_7): Patient lies supine on the table with chin is so raised that lower jaw is at right angle to the table.

Direction and Centring of X-ray Beam: Central rays in midline at the level of angles of the mandible with tube tilted 10° cephalad.

Central ray over midline of body 2" above suprasternal notch at right angles to the film. The patient must hold the breath during exposure.

Distance 90 cm KvP 76 mAs 40

Grid Yes

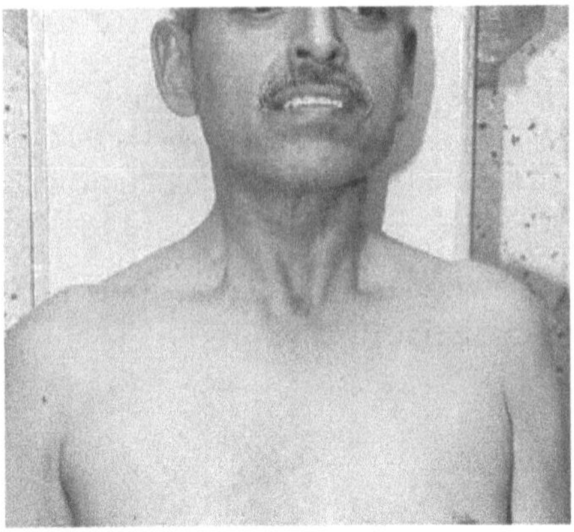

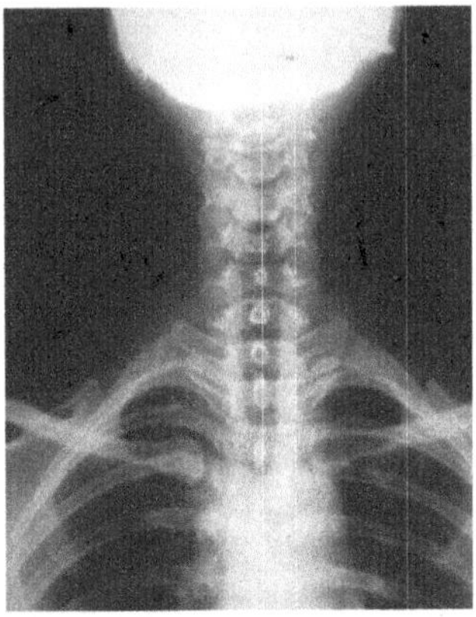

Fig. 2.27: Position of patient for C_{2-7} vertebrae AP view and skiagram for cervical spine AP view

Lateral View for Cervical Spine (C_1-C_7): The patient standing or sitting in true lateral position with one shoulder against the cassette. Both the shoulders should be pulled down as much as possible by asking the patient to hold one sandbag in each hand.

The chin is raised so that the angle of mandible does not obscure upper cervical vertebrae. Head should be kept steady by head clamp. The lower border of film at the level of shoulder and upper border at the level of top of pinna of ear. A long focus film distance of 60" (150 cm) should be used to reduce magnification.

Direction and Centring of X-ray Beam: Central rays just behind the angle of mandible at right angles to the film.

Distance 160 cm KvP 70 mAs 30

Grid No

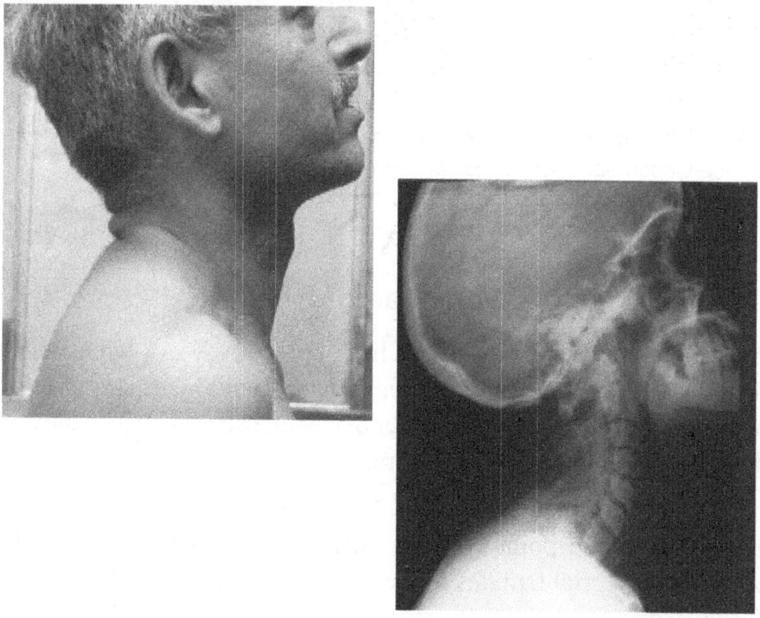

Fig. 2.28: Position of patient for lateral view of cervical spine and skiagram of cervical spine lateral view

Swimmer's Position for Cervicothoracic Vertebrae Lateral View (Lateral-oblique View): Patient is prone on the table. The shoulder of the side to be examined should be close to table top. The other arm to be kept stretched and the arm closer to the film should be stretched in opposite direction to the upper arm, as patient is in swimming position.

Direction and Centring of X-ray Beam: Central rays are focused over most prominent vertebrae or just a cm below it.

15" × 12" size film is kept in bucky.

Distance 90 cm KvP 80 mAs 60

Grid Yes

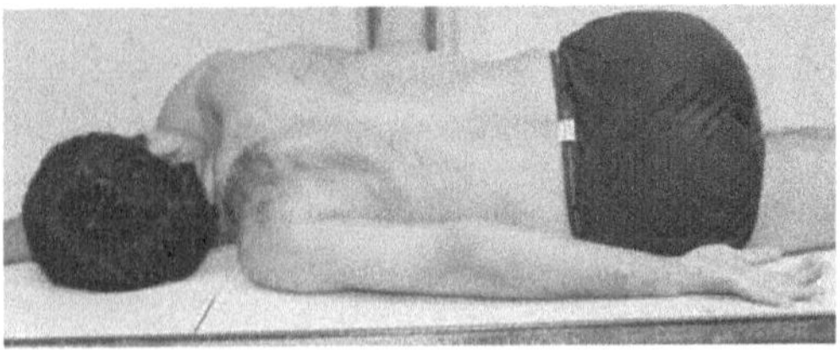

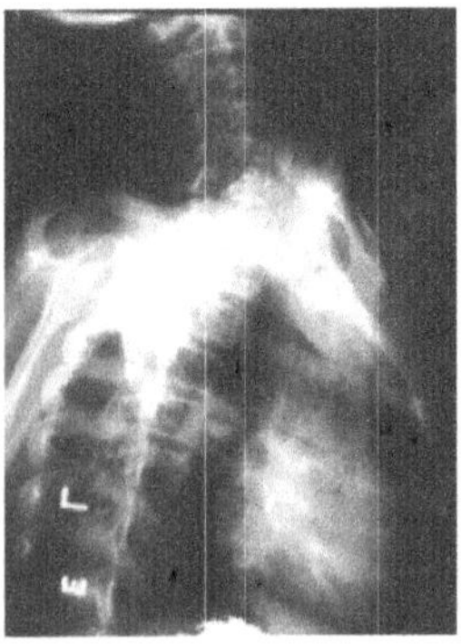

Fig. 2.29: Position of patient for cervical or cervicodorsal spine oblique view and swimmer's view for cervical or cervicodorsal region

Dorsal or Thoracic Vertebrae

Anteroposterior View: Patient lies supine on X-ray table with flexed knee and arms by the side. Patient should lie as straight as possible on the table. Upper border of cassette should be just above the spinous process of C_7 vertebra.

Direction and Centring of X-ray Beam: Central rays are aligned over mid point between suprasternal notch and xiphoid process (D_5) at right angles to the film. Patient should hold breath during exposure.

Distance 90 cm KvP 70 mAs 60

Grid Yes

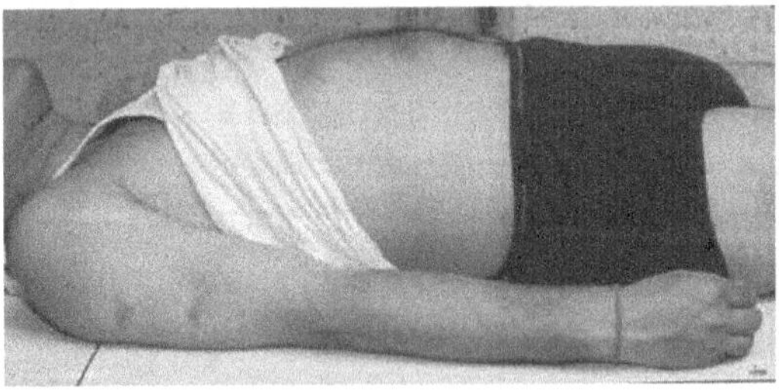

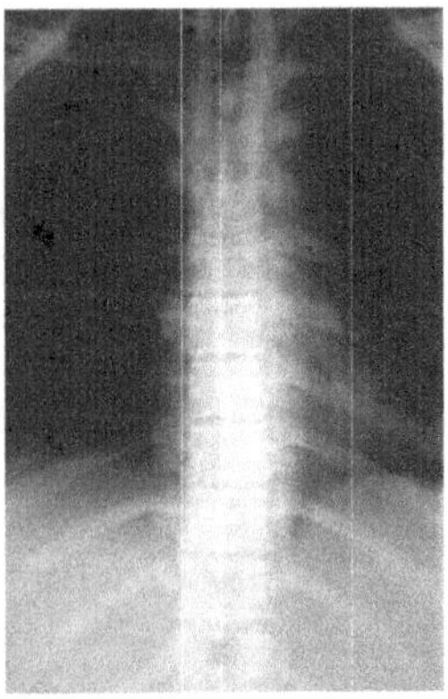

Fig. 2.30: Position of patient for dorsal vertebrae AP view and skiagram for dorsal spine AP view

Lateral View: Patient lies on his side in true lateral position with flexed knees and hands above the head or in front of face. A non opaque pad may be placed under the mid lumbar region.

Direction and Centring of X-ray Beam: Central rays are aligned over D_5 vertebra or through the axilla at right angle to the film and patient should hold the breath during exposure.

Distance 90 cm KvP 80 mAs 100

Grid Yes

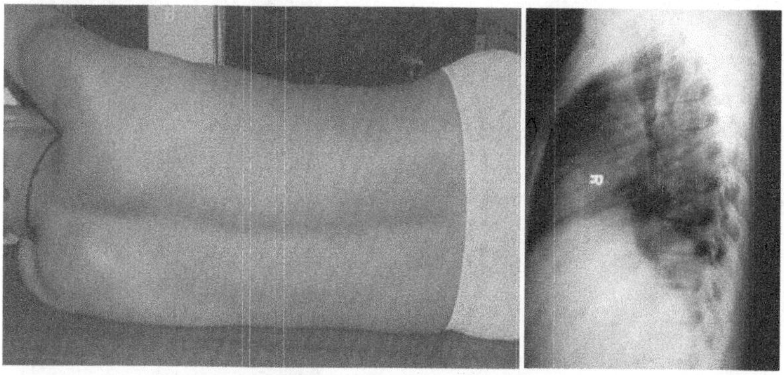

Fig. 2.31: Position of patient for lateral view of dorsal spine and skiagram for dorsal spine lateral view

Cervicodorsal Spine

Oblique Views: Make patient in true lateral position. The arm nearer the film is raised above the head so that the hand touches the opposite ear, the other arm is pulled downward and backward. Then the patient is rotated slightly backwards so that his back is at an angle of 20-30° to the table.

Direction and Centring of X-ray Beam: Central rays at the level of axilla just in front of arm away from the film and at right angles. Patient should hold the breath during exposure (see position for swimmer's view).

Dorsolumbar Vertebrae

Anteroposterior (AP) View: The patient lies supine with knee and hip extended. Sole of feet rest on the table.

Direction and Centring of X-ray Beam: Central rays to the midline at the level of L_1 perpendicular to the film.

Distance 90 cm   KvP 80   mAs 80

Grid Yes

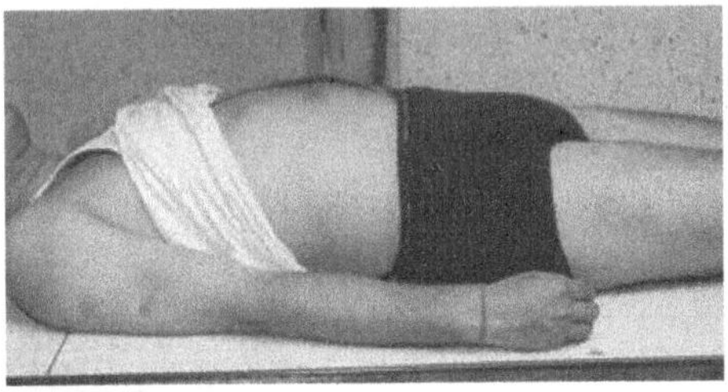

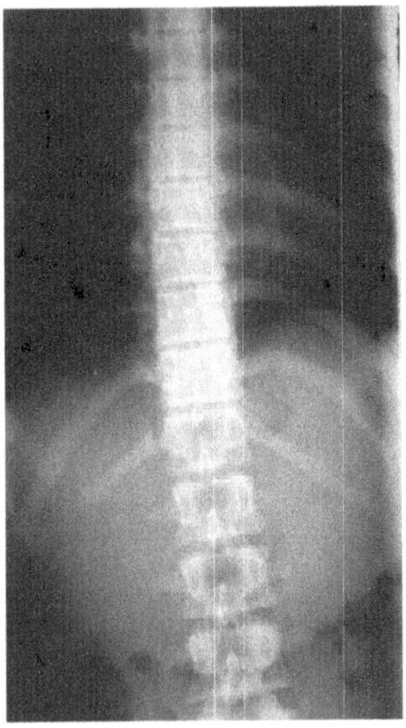

Fig. 2.32: Position of the patient for dorsolumbar AP view and skiagram for dorsolumbar spine AP view

Lateral View: The patient lies on his side with flexed knees. Small pads are placed under the wrist and shoulder to maintain spine parallel with the table.

Direction and Centring of X-ray Beam: Central rays are aligned 3" anterior to spinous process at the level of L_1 at right angle to film.

Distance 90 cm KvP 80 mAs 160

Grid Yes

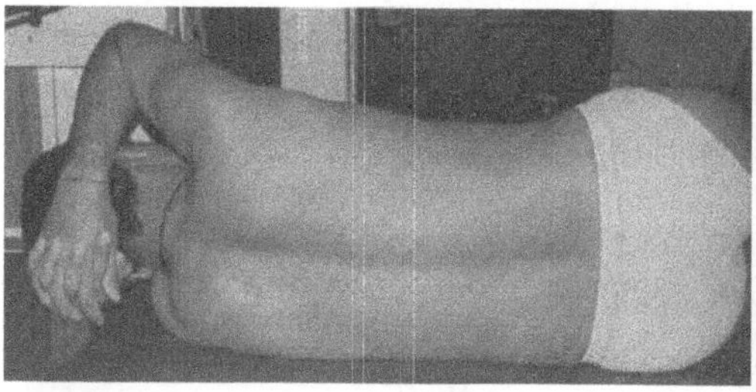

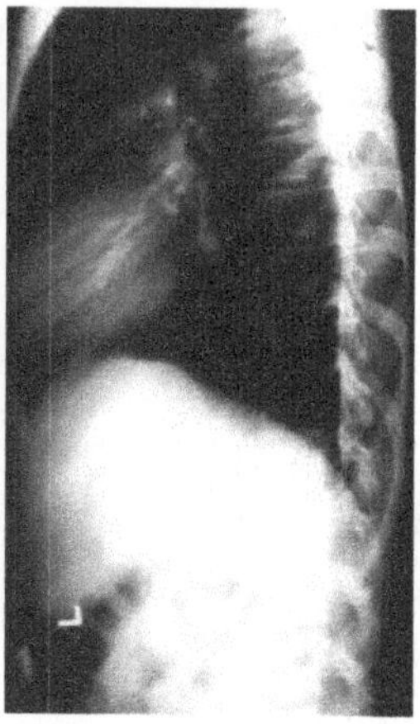

Fig. 2.33: Position of patient for lateral view dorsolateral vertebrae and skiagram showing lateral view dorsolumbar (DL) spine

Lumbar Vertebrae

Anteroposterior View: Patient lies supine on table with knees and hips are flexed. Soles of feet must rest on table to reduce lumbar lordosis. Patient is lying with midline of body as straight as possible.

Direction and Centring of X-ray Beam: Central rays at the level of subcostal margin (over L_3) at right angles to the film.

Distance 90 cm KvP 70 mAs 80

Grid Yes

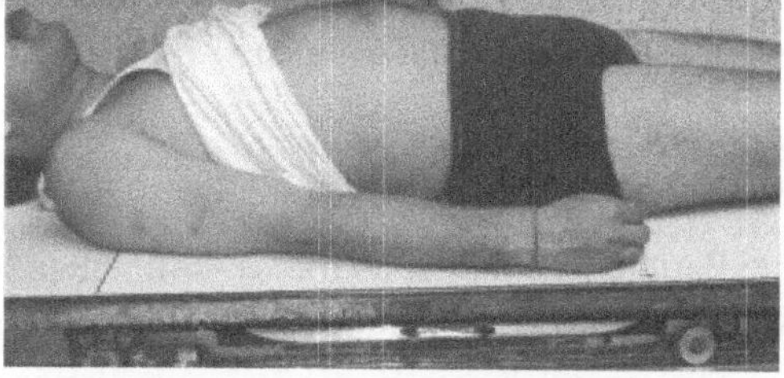

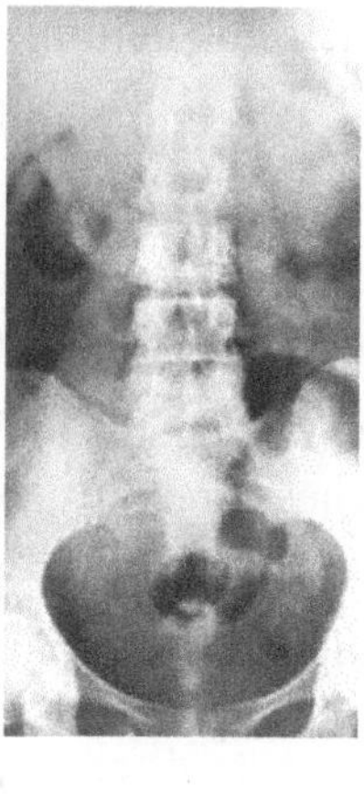

Fig. 2.34: Position of patient for lumbar spine AP view and skiagram showing lumbar spine in AP view

Lateral View: The patient is lying in lateral position, with knees flexed and both hands above the head or in front of face. Patient should be in true lateral position and body is parallel to the table.

Direction and Centring of X-ray Beam: Central rays are aligned to the level of lower costal margin 2-3" anterior to L^3 spinous process at right angles to the film.

Distance 90 cm KvP 80 mAs 160

Grid Yes

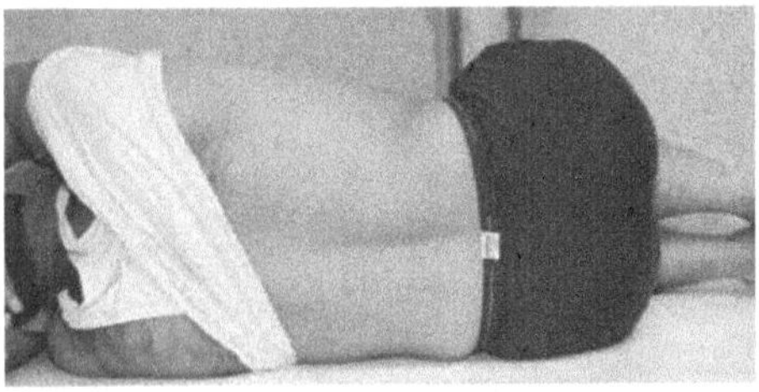

Fig. 2.35a: Position of patient for lumbar vertebrae in lateral view

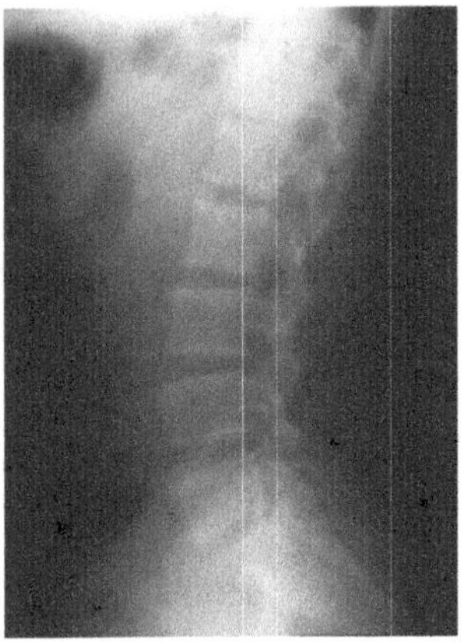

Fig. 2.35b: Skiagram for lateral view lumbar vertebrae

Oblique View: From AP position, rotate the patient about 45° to each side in turn.

Direction and Centring of X-ray Beam: Central rays are aligned to spine at the level of lower costal margin.

Lumbosacral Vertebrae

Anteroposterior View: Patient lies supine as for AP lumbar spine. Knees and hips are extended with sole of feet on the table.

Direction and Centring of X-ray Beam: Central rays are aligned in midline at the level of anterior superior iliac spine with tube angled 15-20° toward the head.

Distance 90 cm KvP 82 mAs 100

Grid Yes

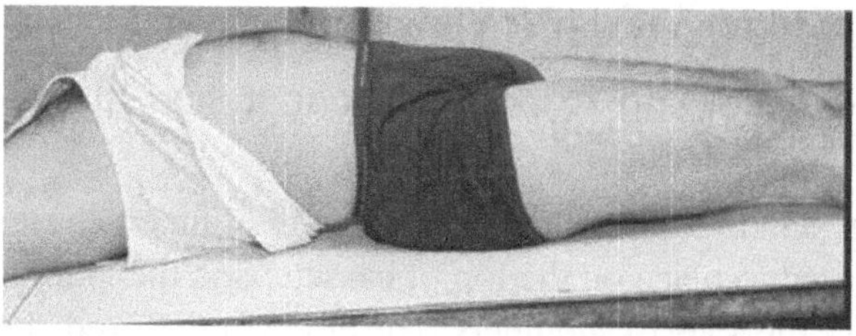

Fig. 2.36: Position of patient for LS spine AP view lumbar and lumbosacral spine AP as seen in Figure 2.34

Lateral View: Patient lying in true lateral position as for lumbar spine. Centre at 3" anterior to spinous process of L_5 vertebra at right angles to the film.

Distance 90 cm KvP 90 mAs 200

Grid Yes

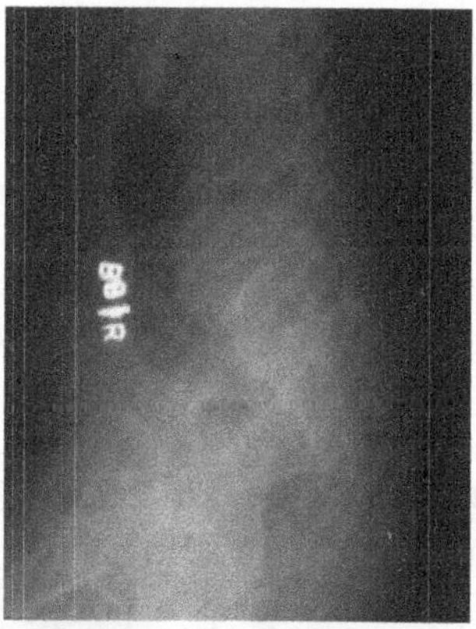

Fig. 2.37: Patient's position can be seen as in Figure 2.35 and skiagram showing lumbosacral spine in lateral view

Oblique View: Patient in the same position as for oblique lumbar spine.

Direction and Centring of X-ray Beam: Centre 2" medial to anterior superior iliac spine with central ray directed 10° to the head.

Distance 90 cm KvP 80 mAs 120

CHEST

Posteroanterior View (PA View)

Film size according to patient's chest size but usually 15" × 12" size.

Patient stands erect with chest against the film on chest stand. Chin is raised to place on the top of cassette and the latter should be 2" above the level of shoulders. The elbows are flexed, the back of hands placed on the hips and elbows are pushed forward, till both the shoulders touches the film. Care is to be taken to see that the patient does not raise his shoulders while bringing them forward towards the cassette.

Direction and Centring of X-ray Beam: Central ray is aligned at D_4–D_5 vertebra level in midline at right angle to film. This point corresponds to midway between the tip of spinous processes of 7th cervical vertebra and mid point of a line joining the lower borders of scapulae. Patient should hold the breath after taking full inspiration during exposure. To minimise the cardiac magnification, FFD should be maintained at 6′ distance and this technique is called as "Teleroentgenogram".

Distance 6′ KvP 60-65 mAs 10-16

Grid No

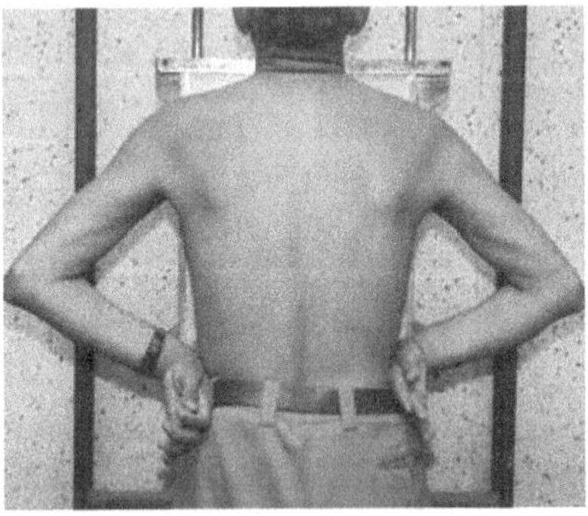

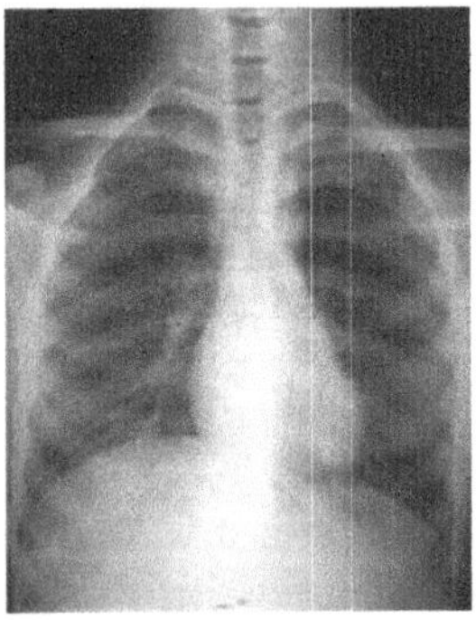

Fig. 2.38: Position of patient for PA view chest and skiagram showing chest PA teleroentgenogram

Anteroposterior (AP) View: Can be done in erect or supine position when patient cannot stand or not conscious or not cooperative, care should be taken to see that the film is high enough to include the apices of the lungs, i.e., top of the film should not be >1" below the occipital protuberance. The shoulders are to be brought forward with hands on hips.

Direction and Centring of X-ray Film: Central ray are passed 2.5 cm below the suprasternal notch at right angles to the film and patient should hold the breath after full inspiration during exposure.

Distance 90 cm KvP 72 mAs 40

Grid Yes

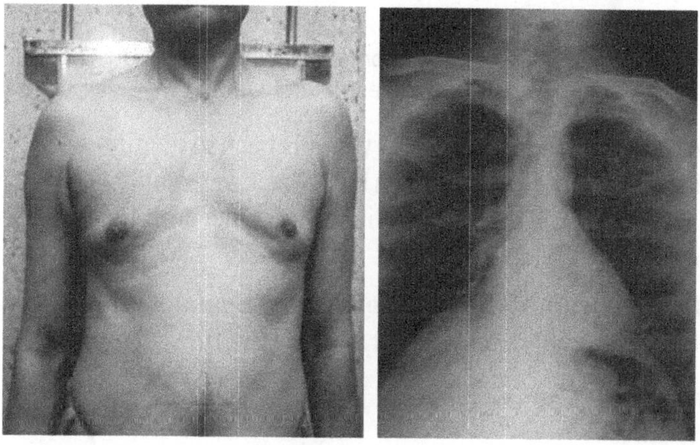

Fig. 2.39: Position of patient for AP view of chest and skiagram for chest AP view

Lateral Views (Right or Left): From PA position, the patient is rotated 90° such that the affected side is in contact with the film in true lateral position. Both the arms are raised straight above the head and the axilla is placed against the cassette. The cassette is so adjusted to include the apices and lung lobes including the posterior costophrenic recess.

Direction and Centring of X-ray Film: Centre through axilla at the level of D_5 at right angles to the film. Patient should hold breath on inspiration during exposure.

Film size 15" × 12" or according to body built.

Distance 90 cm KvP 70 mAs 40

Grid No

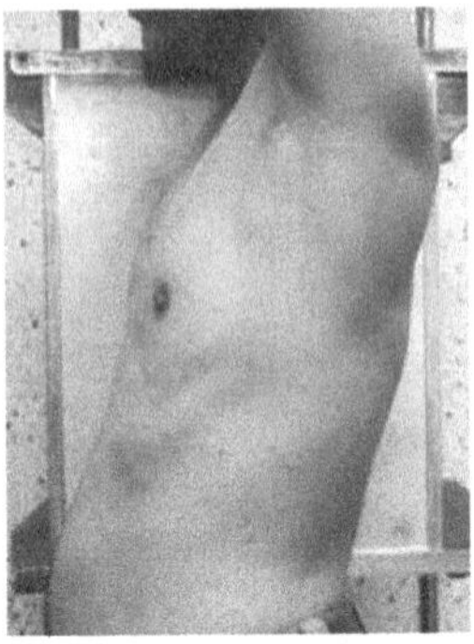

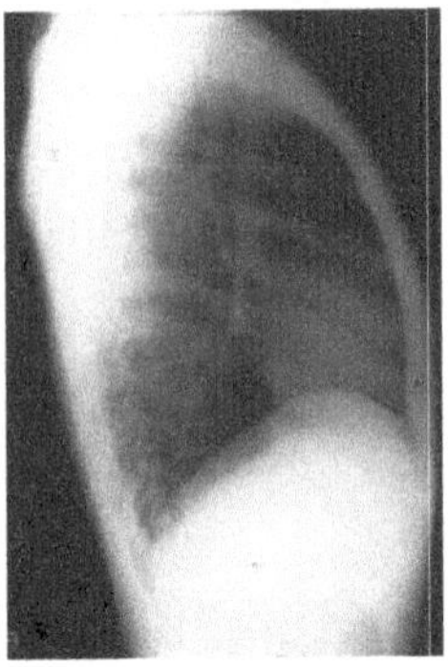

Fig. 2.40: Position of patient for lateral view chest and skiagram showing chest lateral view

Apicogram: Patient is erect with his back to the film and about 12" (30 cm) in front of it. He then bends backward until his shoulders rest on the film. Back of both hands are placed on both hips and elbows pushed backward.

Direction and Centring of X-ray Beam: Central rays is directed to sternal notch at right angle to the film.

Film size 15" × 12" or 12" × 12"

Distance 160 cm KvP 80 mAs 40

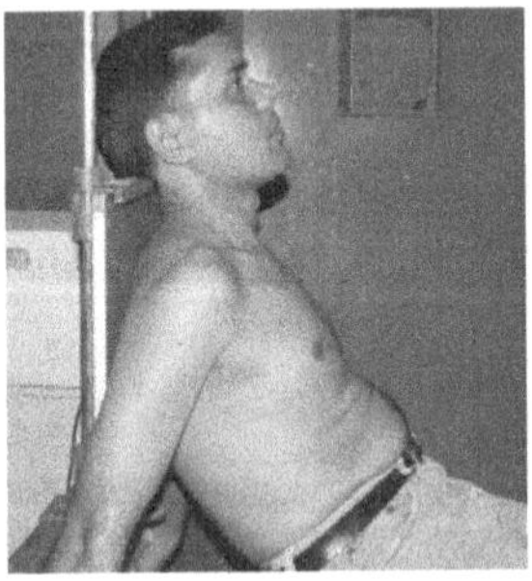

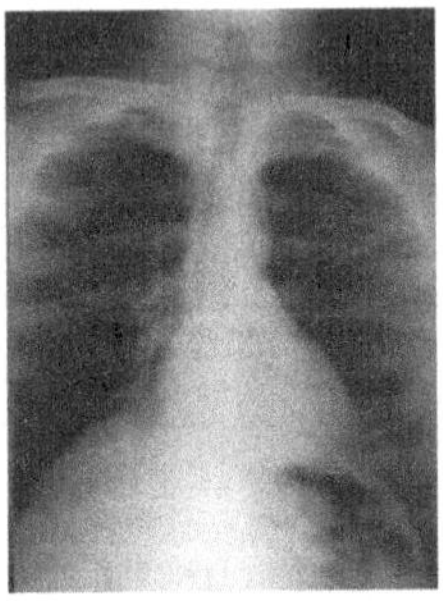

Fig. 2.41: Position of patient for apicogram and skiagram showing chest apical view

Lordotic View: Patient is erect facing the cassette with chin is raised and placed on top of cassette. The patient then grabs the chest stand or the film support and bends backward from the waist approx 30°.

Direction and Centring of X-ray Beam: Central rays are aligned to D_5 level at right angle to film.

Distance 160 cm KvP 80 mAs 40

Grid No

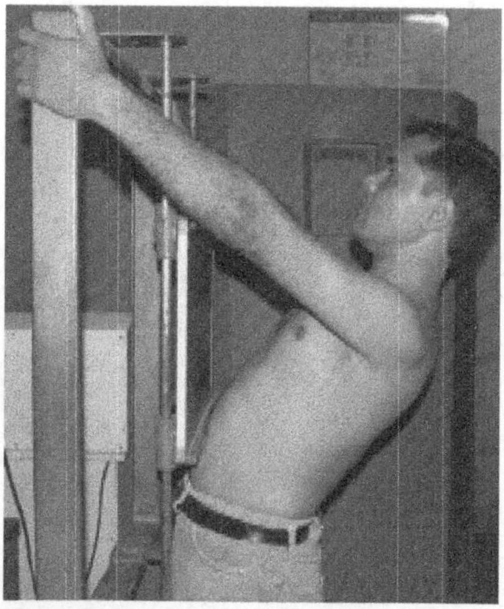

Fig. 2.42: Position of patient for lordotic view

Lateral Decubitus: Position is required when the patient is too ill to stand erect. The patient lies on the affected side to demonstrate fluid in the pleural cavity or on the non-affected side to demonstrate

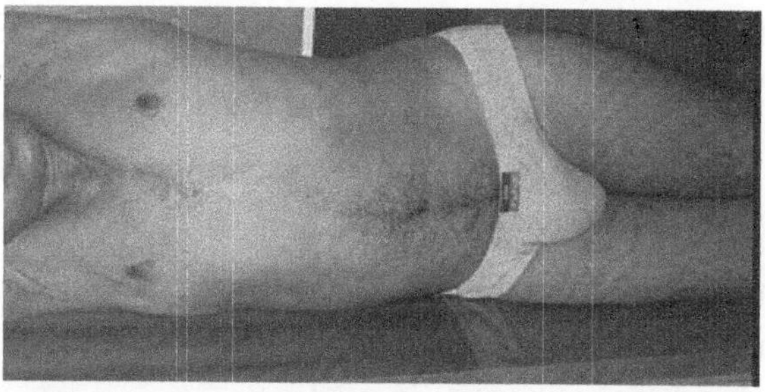

Fig. 2.43: Position of patient for lateral decubitus position

air in the pleural cavity. The patient is kept in true lateral position with both arms straight above the head to avoid superimposition of lung. The cassette is placed vertically behind or in front of the patient.

Direction and Centring of X-ray Beam: Centre are made to the cassette using a horizontal beam. Patient hold his breath after full inspiration during exposure.

Distance 90 cm KvP 80 mAs 40

Reverse Lordotic View: The patient stands erect with his back towards the film. Both hands are kept on hips and the patient leans backwards slightly until the shoulder are in contact with the cassette. The cassette should be so positioned that its upper border is almost at the level of external occipital protuberance of skull.

Centre to xiphisternum with tube angled 30° cephalad.

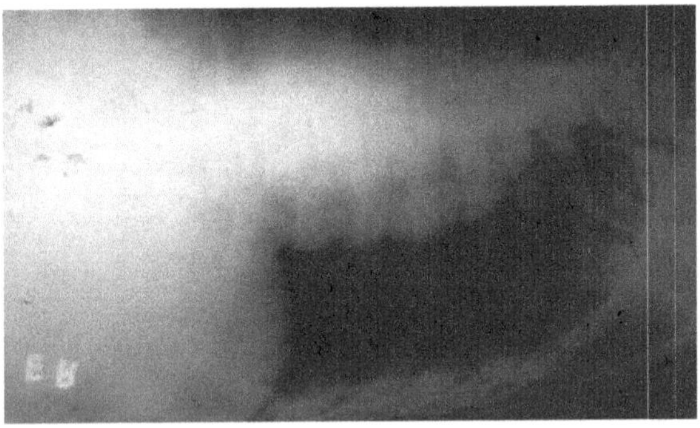

Fig. 2.44: Skiagram for lateral decubitus position

Upper Rib (9 Pairs)

Posteroanterior View: Patient is in erect posture and faces the cassette with chin raised and placed on top of the cassette which should be 2" above the level of shoulders. The elbows are flexed, hands are placed on hips and elbows pushed forward till both the shoulders touch the cassette.

Direction and Centring of X-ray Beam: Central ray over dorsal 5th vertebra, at right angle to the film. Patient holds breath on inspiration during exposure.

Distance 90 cm KvP 72 mAs 40

Grid Yes

Anteroposterior View: Patient erect or supine in true AP position with his back against the film. Shoulders, arms and elbows should be well forward with back of hands on hip.

Direction and Centring of X-ray Beam: Central rays are directed to the level of sternal angle at right angles to film and patient holds respiration during exposure.

Oblique View: For left ribs, left posterior oblique or a right anterior oblique view for right ribs are taken. For the right ribs, right posterior oblique or a left anterior oblique view is taken. The patient is rotated 45° to the right for first oblique film and then to the left for second oblique view. Both hands should be placed on head.

Direction and Centring of X-ray Beam: Central rays are focused over sternum at the level of a line joining the axillae at right angles to the film. Patient should hold the respiration during exposure.

Lower Ribs

Anteroposterior View: This view will show maximum no. of ribs under the diaphragm.

Oblique View: From anteroposterior position, patient is rotated 45° to the affected side. The film is placed with its lower border just below the lower costal margin.

Direction and Centring of X-ray Beam: Central rays in the mid clavicular line for the side being examined at the level of lower costal margin at right angles to the film. Patient should hold the breath in expiration.

Sternum

Posteroanterior View: Patient stands or lies facing the cassette with sternum in midline of cassette. Shoulder should touch the film with arms at sides.

Direction and Centring of X-ray Beam: Central rays are aligned at the level of L_5, 3-4" lateral to spine with tube angled 30° towards the midline of body. Patient should hold respiration during exposure.

Distance 160 cm KvP 72 mAs 60

Grid No

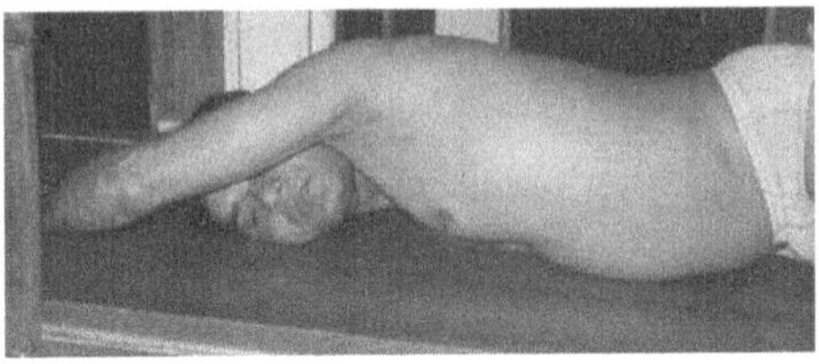

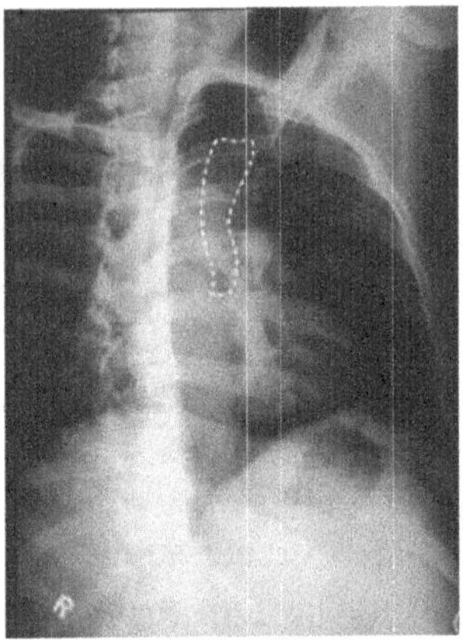

Fig. 2.45: Position of patient for sternum AP view and skiagram showing sternum AP view

Oblique View: Patient prone on table or standing with chest against film of erect posture is raised then the patient is notched of an angle of 35° to the film so that sternum is no longer superimposed by dorsal vertebrae.

Direction and Centring of X-ray Beam: Central rays aligned 2" caudal to level of sternal notch above 4" away from midline, on the side further from the cassette and thus directly through sternum at right angle to the film.

Lateral View: Patient is in true lateral position either on table or in erect position. The shoulders are drawn well back and hands clasped behind the back. Chin is slightly raised.

Direction and Centring of X-ray Beam: Central rays are aligned to pass to sternal angle over front of chest, at right angles to the film. Patient should hold the respiration during exposure.

HEART AND GREAT VESSELS

Posteroanterior (PA) View for Chest

- PA chest is necessary as in cases of PA view chest for lungs.
- Right anterior oblique view—Patient is erect facing the cassette. Patient is rotated from PA position to make 45° angle with film. Left shoulder is away from the film and right shoulder in contact with film. Right arm is kept behind patient's back or at the side and left arm is raised forwards and upwards with hand resting on head.

Direction and Centring of X-ray Beam: Central rays are aligned over left scapula at the level of D_5 at right angles to the film. Patient should hold breath after full inspiration during exposure.

Distance 90 cm KvP 72 mAs 40

Grid No

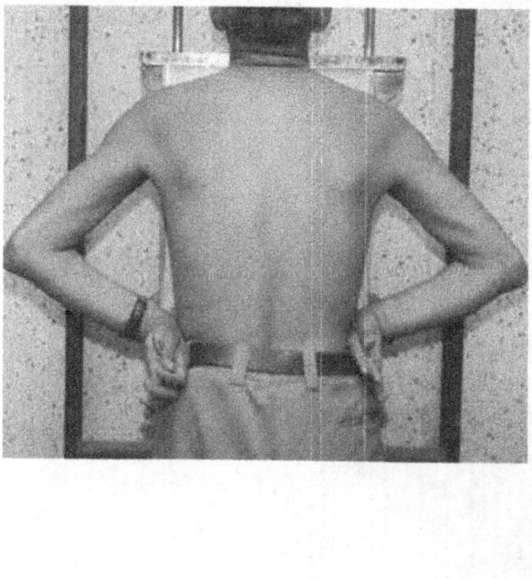

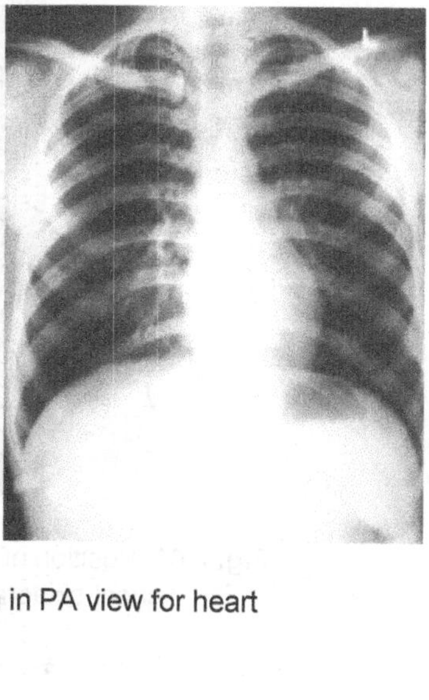

Fig. 2.46: Chest skiagram in PA view for heart

Oblique View: It could be left anterior/posterior or Rt anterior/posterior in positioning process is same except the patient is rotated to the side required for viewing.

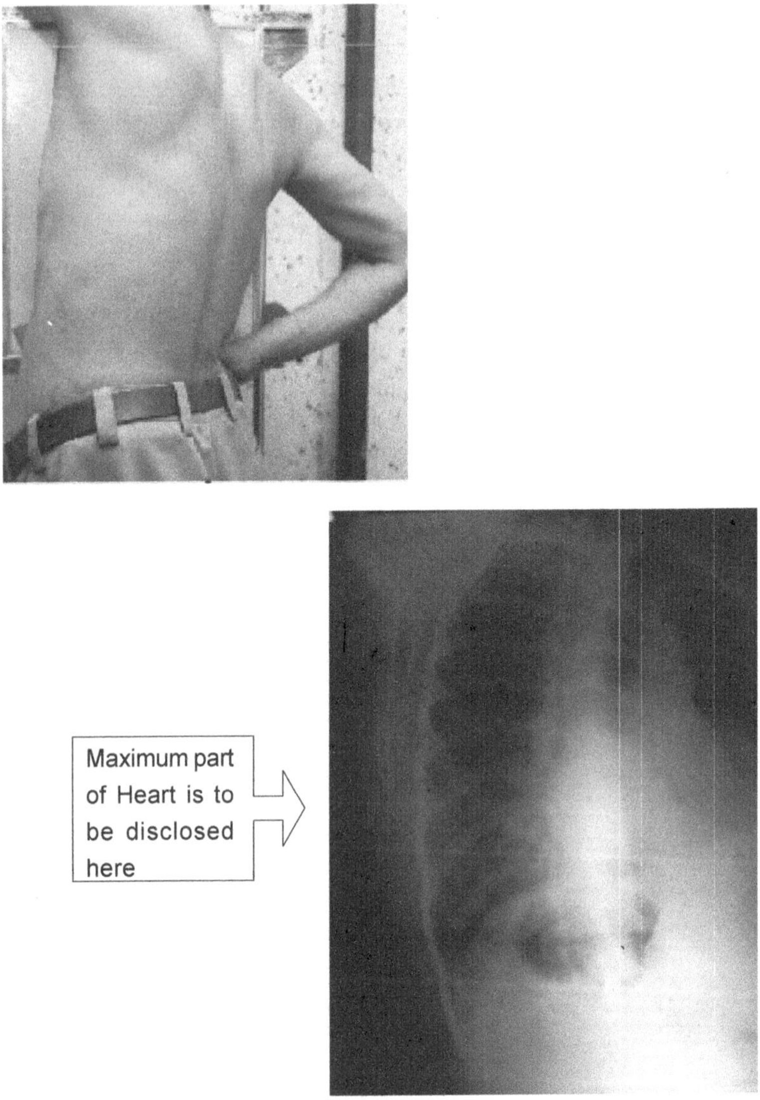

Fig. 2.47: Position of patient in LAO view and chest skiagram in LAO view

Pharynx and Larynx

Pharynx Anatomy—Pharynx extends from the base of skull to the cricoid cartilage and is situated behind the nose, mouth and upper part of throat. It is divided into 3 parts:

1. *Nasopharynx*—It lies behind the nose and above the soft palate. It communicates with the middle ears via eustachian tube.
2. *Oropharynx*—It lies behind the mouth and extends from the soft palate to the epiglottis.
3. *Laryngopharynx*—It extends from upper border of epiglottis to the lower border of cricoid cartilage where it becomes continuous with the esophagus.

Lateral View for Nasopharynx (Post nasal space): Patient sits or stands in true lateral position with close to cassette and immobilised raised chin. The upper border of cassette is placed at the level of glabella. Beam is collimated to avoid exposure to thyroid, the patient is asked to breath in deeply through nose so that post nasal space is filled with air.

Direction and Centring of X-ray Beam: Central rays are aligned to lower border of zygoma. Exposure is made with patient holding his breath after deep inspiration.

Larynx: Anatomy of larynx is composed of a ring of cartilaginous structures of which thyroid, cricoid and arytenoid cartilages are important. The upper opening of larynx is in floor of pharynx and it continues into the trachea at its lower end. The main function of larynx is to act as a valvular sphincter guarding the entry into pulmonary air tract. Production of sound is the main function.

Lateral View: Patient stands or sits with one shoulder against the cassette. The head should be in true lateral position. The chin is raised, head and the shoulders are lowered as much as possible. Upper border of the cassette should be at the level of top of pinna of ear.

Direction and Centring of the X-ray Beam: Centre 2" posterior to anterior border of neck at the level of laryngeal prominence. Central rays are aligned at right angles to the film. Exposure is made on suspended deep respiration.

Thoracic Inlet: Thoracic inlet is bounded posteriorly by the first thoracic vertebra, anteriorly by manubrium sterni and laterally by 1st ribs. Trachea, esophagus, vessels and nerves pass through thoracic inlet.

Anteroposterior View: The patient lies supine on the table with chin raised with body's coronal plane parallel to table top and median sagittal plane perpendicular to the table. Exposure may be made either on suspended full inspiration or preferably with the patient performing. "Valsalva technique" (Patient is asked to take in deep breath and then to blow out forcibly while mouth keeping in closed position) and pinching the nose with thumb and index finger.

Direction and Centring of X-ray Beam: Central rays are allowed to pass through sternal notch at right angles to the film.

Lateral View: Patient stands erect in a true lateral position with the chin slightly raised. Both hands should be clasped behind the back and shoulders forced as far back as possible.

Direction and Centring of X-ray Beam: Central rays are aligned to sternal notch at right angles to the film on full inspiration.

VIEW FOR FOREIGN BODY ESOPHAGUS AND LEFT ATRIAL ENLARGEMENT

Anatomy: The esophagus commences over median vertical plane at the level of C_6 and extends downward to the level of D_{11} when it continues with stomach. At the level of D_{10}, it passes slightly to the left of median vertical plane. Esophagus lies behind the heart and in front of dorsal vertebrae.

Skiagrams are taken in anteroposterior, true lateral and both oblique views as in skiagrams of chest. Any radio-opaque foreign body are identified by their size and shape. In adults, most common foreign bodies are denture fishbone or chickenbone. In children most common foreign body are small coins, screws and nails etc.

Direction and Centring of X-ray Beam: Central rays as in skiagram of chest.

Exposure same as in skiagram of chest.

DIAPHRAGM

Diaphragm is a fibromuscular division between chest and abdomen. Diaphragm is attached by muscle and tendinous fibres to bony skeleton, the spine posteriorly, the ribs laterally and the sternum anteriorly. Although the diaphragm functions as single muscle, it is customary to divide it into right and left leaf or cupola. The diaphragm forms part of respiratory mechanism. It is lowered on inspiration and elevated on expiration. In an erect PA chest view, upper border of diaphragm is seen at the level of 10th ribs on expiration. Diaphragm is rarely the primary site of pulmonary disease or by phrenic nerve damage. It is also a common site of trauma or may be congenitally deficient. The main purpose of radiographic examination of the diaphragm is the investigation of structure above and below it.

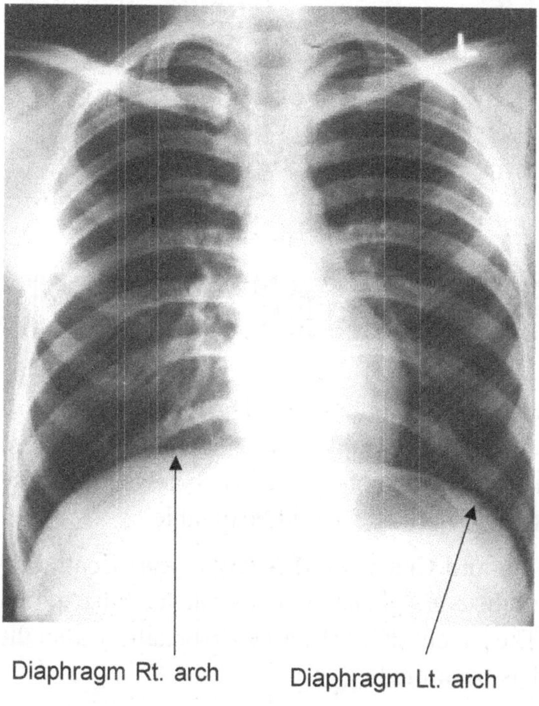

Fig. 2.48: Diaphragm

Posteroanterior View: The patient stands erect facing the cassette which is placed transversely with its lower border at the level of lower costal margin. Patient is asked to keep his hands over his head.

Centring of X-ray Beam: Centre to xiphisternum or middle of film, perpendicular to film.

Lateral View: Patient is erect and in true lateral position, the suspected disease side should be in contact with cassette with patient raising his both hands above the head. Care should be taken to see that upper border of the cassette is at the level of axilla.

Direction and Centring of the X-ray Beam: Central rays through axilla at right angle to film.

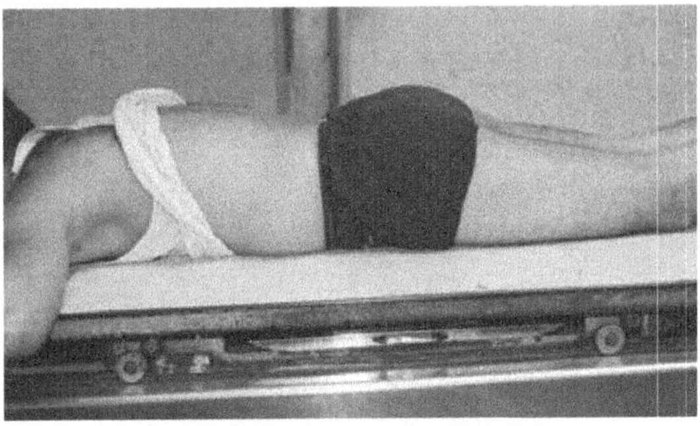

Fig. 2.49: Translateral view

ABDOMEN

Anteroposterior (Supine) View: The patient lies supine on table with knee flexed over a small pillow for comfort. The cassette is so positioned that its lower border is 2.5 cm below the pubic symphysis. Midline of body should be in middle of table.

Direction and Centring of X-ray Beam: Central rays passes through umbilicus at right angles to the film on full expiration during exposure. The patient should be asked to breathe in after the required exposure has been made.

Film size 17" × 14" or according to patient's body built.

Distance 90 cm KvP 72 mAs 80

Grid Yes (moving grid)

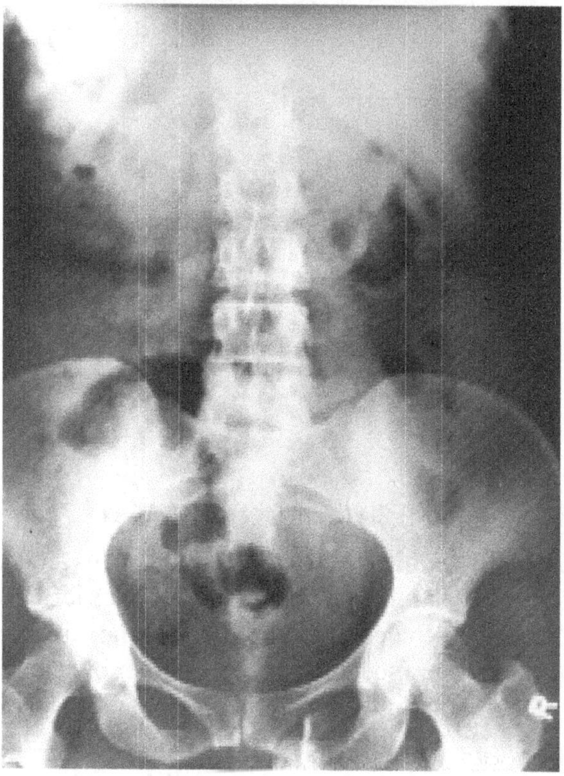

Fig. 2.50: Skiagram for AP abdomen (Supine)

Anteroposterior (Erect) View: The patient stands erect with his back against the bucky. The cassette should be so positioned that in upper border is 5 cm above the xiphisternum to include the diaphragm.

Film size 17" × 14" or according to patient's body built.

Direction and Centring of the X-ray Beam: Central rays passes through middle of cassette just above umbilicus at right angle to film.

Distance 90 cm KvP 80 mAs 80

Grid Yes

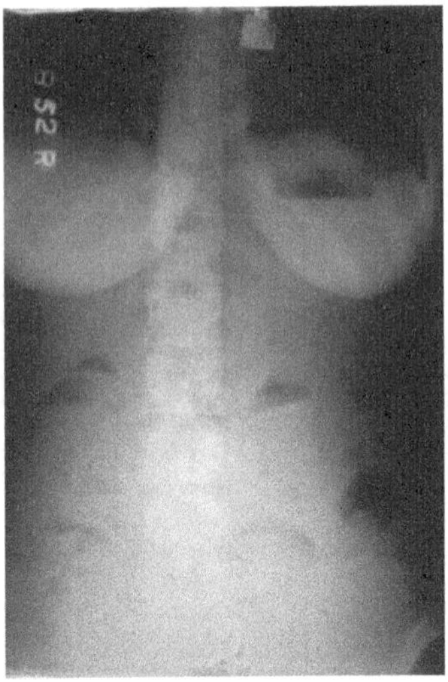

Fig. 2.51: Skiagram for erect abdomen

Left Lateral Decubitus View: Patient lies on his left side with cassette vertically placed in contact with his anterior abdominal wall. The hands are folded and placed above the patient's head. Care should be taken to see that the upper border of cassette is 5.0 cm above the level of xiphisternum so as to include diaphragm.

Direction and Centring of X-ray Beam: Central rays in midline at the middle of cassette at right angles to the film using an horizontal beam.

Film size 15" × 12" or according to patient's body built.

Distance 90 cm KvP 82 mAs 120

Lateral View: The patient is turned to side under examination with hip and knee flexed. The median sagittal plane is parallel to the film. The mid axillary line of body is in midline of the table. Centre of film should be approx 5.0 cm above the highest point of iliac crest. Patient should hold the breath after full expiration during exposure.

URINARY TRACT AND RETROPERITONEAL STRUCTURES

Anteroposterior (KUB)/Scout Film of Abdomen: Patient lies supine with centre of body in line of centre of the table. The lower border of cassette should be 2.5 cm below the pubic symphysis. Centre of cassette should be at about the level of lower costal margin in mid axillary line and upper edge of cassette is at the level of xiphisternum.

Direction and Centring of the X-ray Beam: Central rays is directed vertically to the centre of the film. Patient is instructed to hold breath after full expiration during exposure.

Film size 17" × 14" or according to patient's body built.

Distance 90 cm KvP 72 mAs 80

Grid Yes

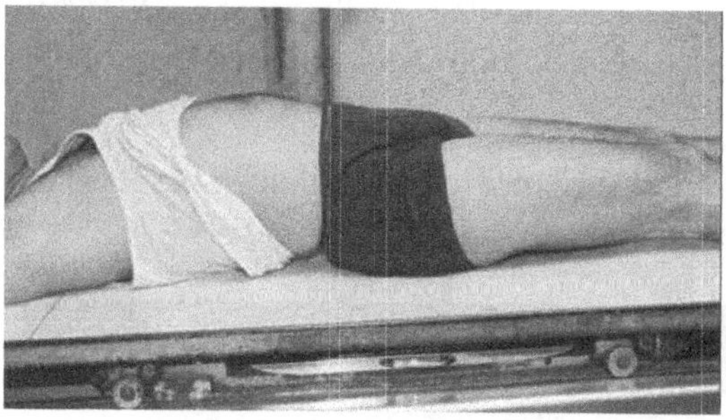

Fig. 2.52a: Position of patient for supine/ scout abdomen

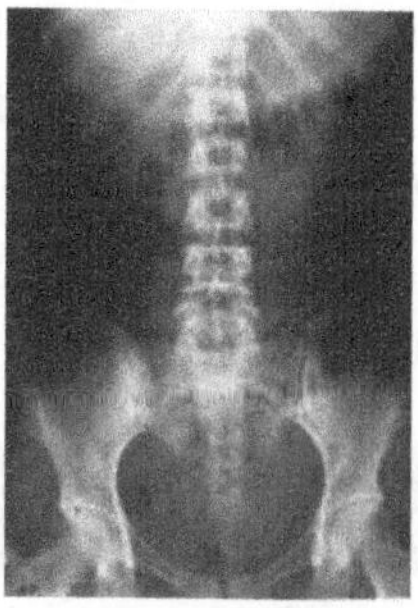

Fig. 2.52b: Supine for KUB or scout film

Posterior Oblique (for Urinary Bladder) View: Patient in supine position is rotated through 30° with point midway between pubic symphysis and anterior superior iliac spine or raised side should be over the midline of the table.

Centring of the X-ray Beam: Central rays 1" (2.5 cm) above the pubic symphysis at right angles to the film.

ANTEROPOSTERIOR (FOR PREGNANCY) VIEW

Film size 17" × 14"

Distance 90 cm KvP 100 mAs 60

(High KV technique)

Patient is advised to empty her urinary bladder before X-ray examination. Patient lies supine on table with centre of the body in midline of the table. Feel the pubic symphysis and lower border of cassette must be 1-1.5" below the pubic symphysis.

Direction and Centring of the X-ray Beam: Central rays are directed vertically at the centre of the film. Patient is asked to hold breath after full expiration during exposure.

ANTEROPOSTERIOR VIEW FOR LIVER

Anteroposterior (for Liver) View: Patient lies supine. A 15" × 12" cassette is used transversely with its lower border at the level of iliac crest.

Centring of X-ray Beam: Centre in the midline at the level of midline of cassette at right angle to the film.

ANTEROPOSTERIOR VIEW FOR SPLEEN

Anteroposterior (Spleen) View: The patient lies supine. A 10" × 12" cassette is used with its lower border at the level of lower costal margin.

Centring of X-ray Beam: Centre in the mid clavicular line at the level of middle of cassette.

UPPER EXTREMITY

Humerus Anteroposterior (AP) View

Positioning of Patient: Patient supine on the table with the unaffected shoulder raised and supported on sandbags to bring the shoulder and arm of the side being examined into the contact with cassette. The arm is adjusted to make sure that the medial and lateral epicondyles of the humerus are equidistant from the film. To reduce the risk of movement a sandbag should be placed over the palm of the hand and the exposure made during arrested respiration.

Film size 15" × 6"

Direction and Centring of X-ray Beam: The vertical central ray is directed to a point midway between the shoulder and elbow joint.

Distance 90 cm KvP 54 mAs 12

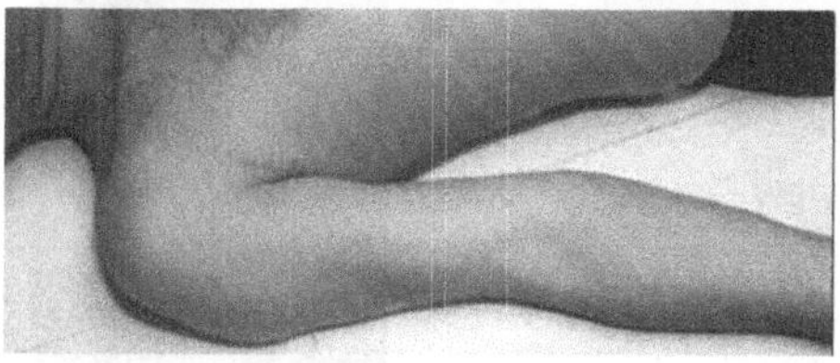

↑ Position of humerus AP view

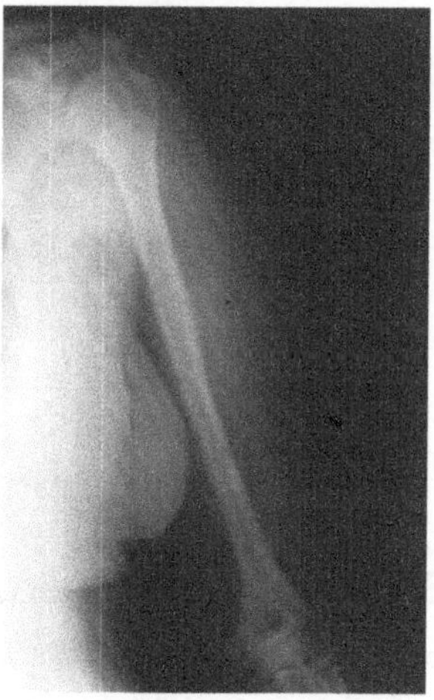

Fig. 2.53: Anteroposterior (AP) view humerus

Humerus Lateral View

Positioning of Patient: From the position for the anteroposterior projection, the elbow is flexed to 90°, the arm abducted and then medially rotated through 90° to bring the medial aspect of the arm, elbow and forearm into contact with the table. A film, large enough to include the shoulder and elbow joints is placed under the arm. The epicondyles of humerus should be superimposed vertically.

Film size 15" × 6"

Direction and Centring of X-ray Beam: The vertical central ray is directed to a point midway between the shoulder and elbow joint.

Distance 90 cm KvP 54 mAs 12

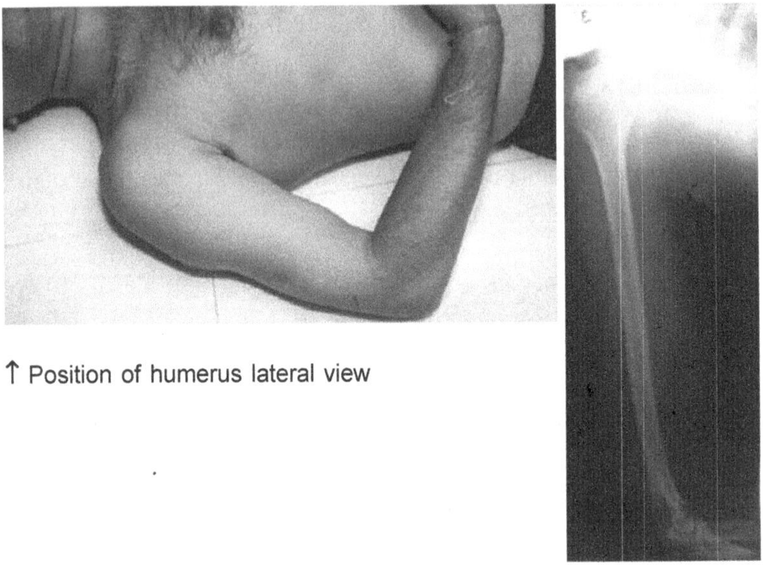

↑ Position of humerus lateral view

Fig. 2.54: Lateral view of humerus or upper arm

Shoulder Joint Anteroposterior View

Positioning of Patient: AP projection is taken in either with the patient supine on the X-ray table or erect, sitting, standing, with the back against a vertical bucky. The patient faces the X-ray tube and is then rotated towards the affected side to bring the posterior aspect of affect shoulder into contact with the midline of the table or vertical bucky. The film should be large enough to include the shoulder joint and proximal half of humerus.

Film size 12" × 10"

Direction and Centring of the X-ray Beam: The central rays is directed at right angles to the humerus and centred to the head of the humerus. The exposure is made on arrested respirations.

Distance 90 cm KvP 60 mAs 20

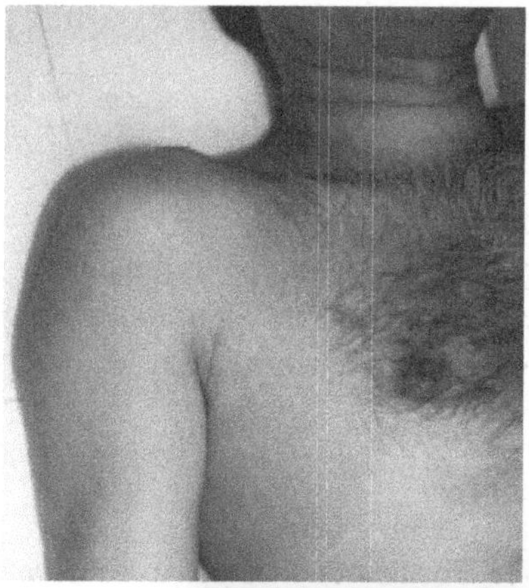

← Position of shoulder joint AP view

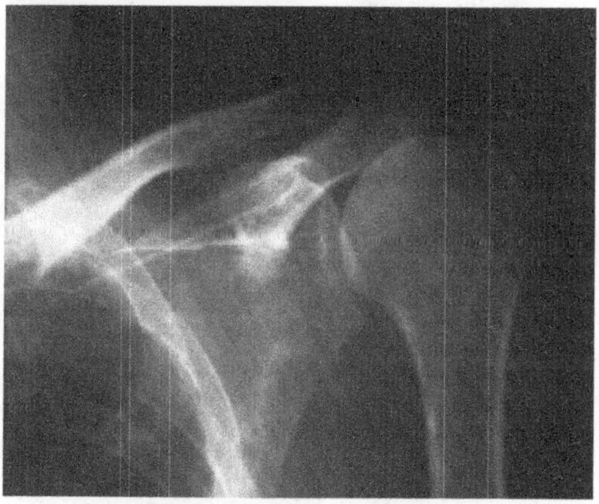

Fig. 2.55: Shoulder in anteroposterior (AP) position

Shoulder Joint Axial View

Positioning of the Patient: The patient stands against a vertical support with the affected arm by the side, supported in partial abduction. The palm of the hand is relaxed facing the trunk so that the line joining the epicondyles of the humerus is at an angle of 45° to the trunk. A film is supported horizontally above the affected shoulder with its centre over the shoulder joint.

Direction and Centring of X-ray Beam: The central ray is vertical, making an angle of 10° to the shaft of the humerus and is directed towards the anterior aspect of head of humerus. Exposure should be taken during arrested respiration.

Distance 90 cm KvP 60 mAs 25

Alternatively, the patient is supine with film supported vertically above the shoulder. The arm rests on the table with palm facing the patient's side and line joining the epicondyles at 45° to the table. The central ray is directed horizontally to anterior part of head of humerus.

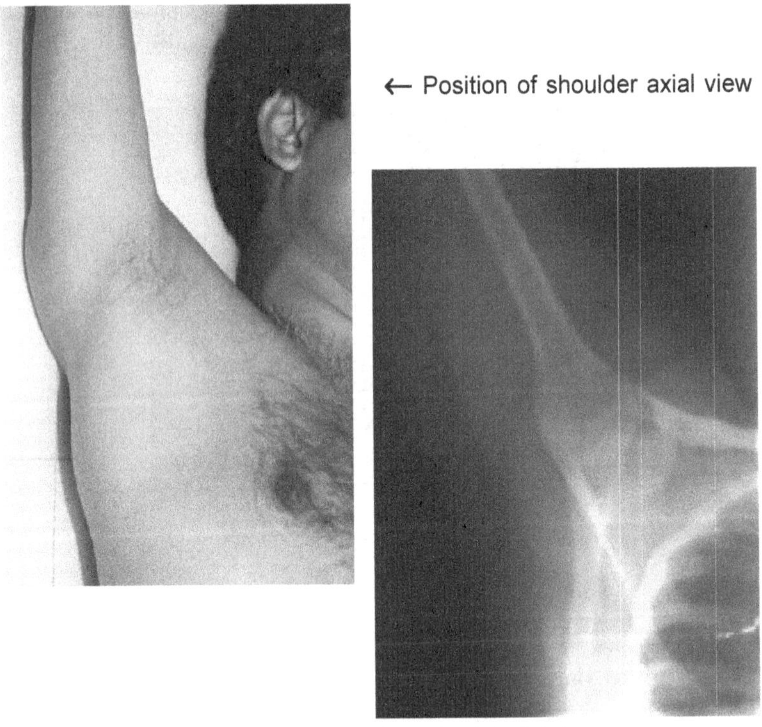

← Position of shoulder axial view

Fig. 2.56: Axial view shoulder joint

Elbow Joint Anteroposterior View

Positioning of the Patient: Patient supine with arm and forearm fully extended so that posterior aspect of entire limb is in contact with table and palm facing upward. The film is placed under the elbow with its centre under the joint and its long axis parallel to the limb. Medial and lateral epicondyles should be equidistant from the film.

Direction and Centring of X-ray Beam: The vertical central ray is directed through the joint space 2.5 cm distal to mid point between the epicondyles of humerus.

Film size 10" × 8"

Distance 90 cm KvP 54 mAs 16

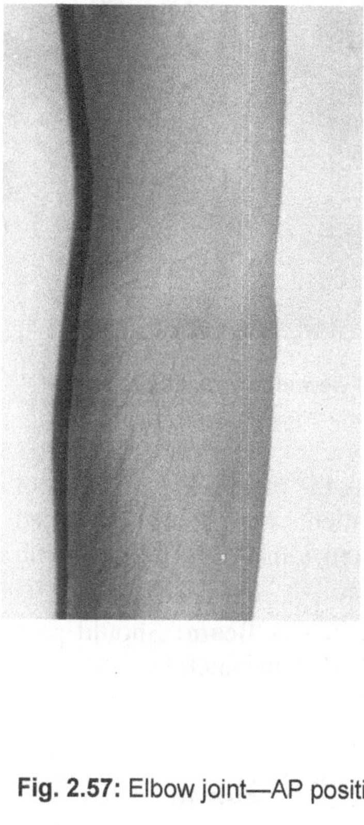

← Position of elbow joint AP view

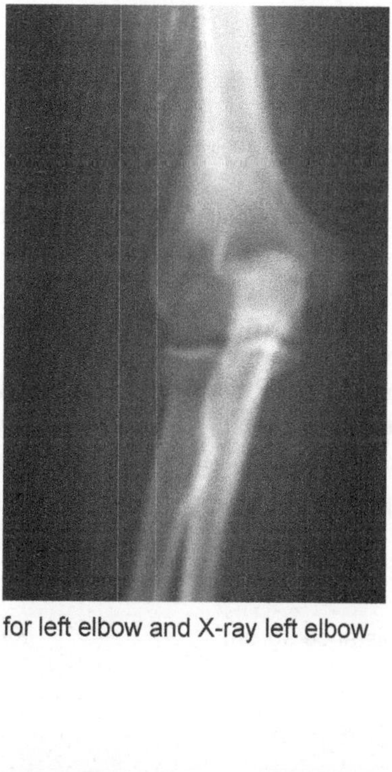

Fig. 2.57: Elbow joint—AP position for left elbow and X-ray left elbow

Elbow Joint Lateral View

Positioning of the Patient: The patient is seated at the side of the table with the arm abducted, the elbow flexed to 90° and palm at 90° to the table. The shoulder should be at the level of elbow and wrist so that medial aspect of limb is in contact with the table.

Direction and Centring of the X-ray Beam: The vertical central ray is directed to the lateral epicondyle of the humerus.

Film size 12" × 10"

Distance 90 cm KvP 52 mAs 16

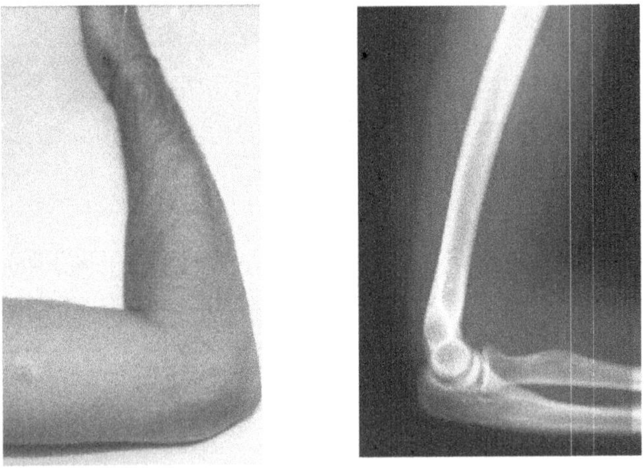

Fig. 2.58: Position of patient for lateral view elbow joint and X-ray of elbow joint in lateral view

Axial View for Elbow Joint: Ask the patient to sit on a stool placed nearer to the X-ray table. Patients arm should be flexed maximum. Rotate forearm until wrist comes in lateral position (thumb up). The tube is rotated by 45 degrees.

Direction and Centring of the X-ray Beam: Should pass through midpoint of both condyles (medial and lateral).

Film size 12" × 10"

Distance 90 cm KvP 52 mAs 16

Forearm Anteroposterior (AP) View

Positioning of Patient: The patient is seated at the side of the table with the arm abducted, the elbow is fully extended and supinated forearm resting on the table. The film should cover both elbow and wrist joints, so that radial and ulnar styloid processes as well as medial and lateral epicondyles of the humerus are equidistant from the film.

Film size 15" × 6"

Direction and Centring of X-ray Beam: The vertical central ray is directed in the midline of the forearm to a point midway between the elbow and wrist.

Distance 90 cm KvP 52 mAs 12

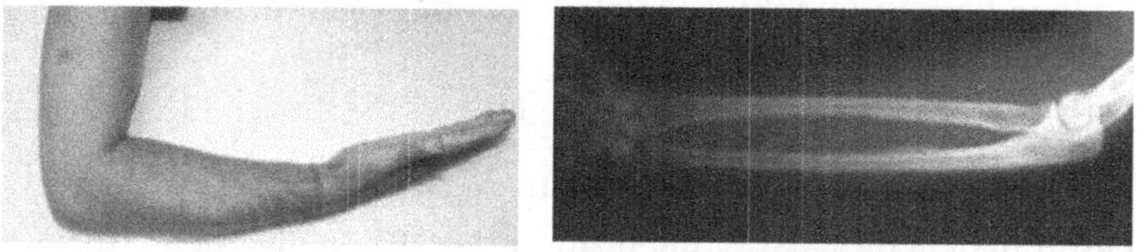

Fig. 2.59: Position for forearm AP view and X-ray of forearm AP view

Forearm Lateral View

Positioning of Patient: From the previous position the elbow is flexed to a right angle and then the humerus medially rotated through 90° to bring the medial aspect of upper arm, elbow, forearm, wrist and hand into contact with table. A film should cover elbow and wrist both the joints.

Film size 15" × 6"

Direction and Centring of the X-ray Beam: The vertical ray is directed to the lateral aspect of the forearm midway between the elbow and wrist.

Distance 90 cm KvP 54 mAs 12

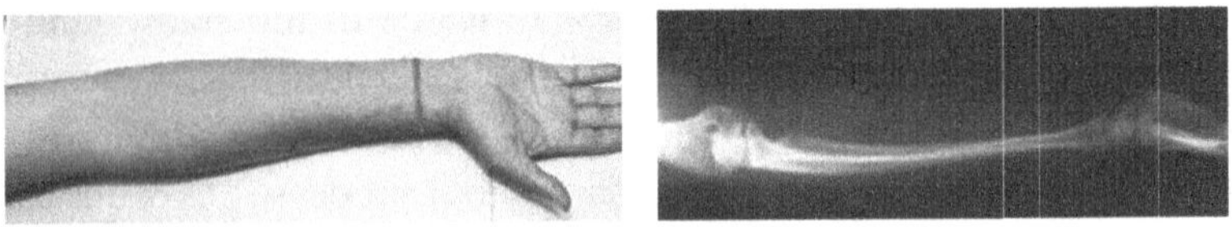

(a) (b)

Fig. 2.60: (a) Position of patient for forearm in lateral view
(b) X-ray of forearm in lateral view

Hand: Anteroposterior (AP) View

Positioning of Patient: The patient is seated with the forearm placed on the table in pronation and the palm with fingers resting on the film. The fingers are separated and extended but relaxed to bring them into close contact with the film. The wrist is adjusted to bring the radial and ulnar styloid processes equidistant from the film and then limb is immobilised with a sandbag over the forearm.

Film size 10" × 8"

Direction and Centring of the X-ray Beam: The vertical central rays is directed to the head of the 3rd metacarpal.

Distance 90 cm KvP 45 mAs 8

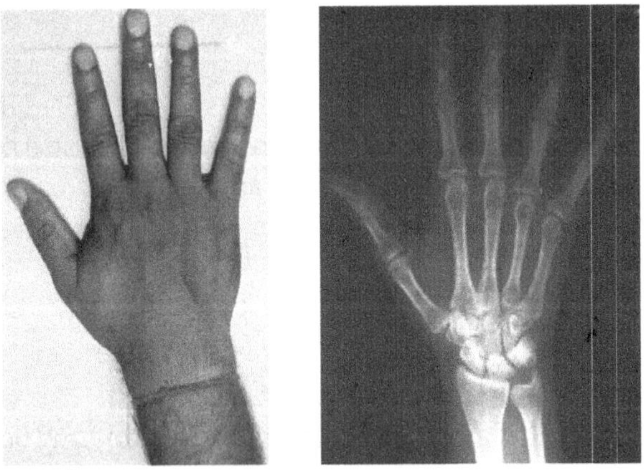

Fig. 2.61: Position of patient for right hand PA view, and X-ray of right hand in PA view

Hand: Anterior Oblique View

Positioning of Patient: From the position of posteroanterior view, the hand is laterally rotated through 45° and supported in this position. The fingers are separated and extended but relaxed with the tips of fingers resting on a non-opaque pad. Alternatively, by slight flexing the fingers so that their tips can rest on the film supporting the hand in an oblique position.

Film size 10" × 8"

Direction and Centring of X-ray Beam: The vertical central ray is directed to the head of 5th metacarpal. The tube angled so that the central ray is directed to the head of 3rd metacarpal.

Distance 90 cm KvP 48 mAs 10

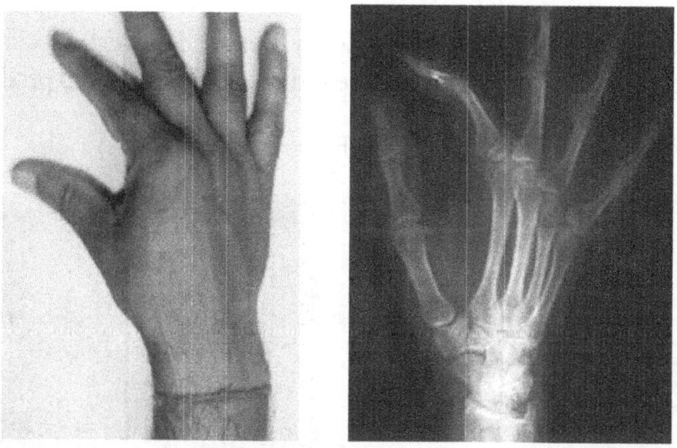

Fig. 2.62: Position of right hand in oblique view and X-ray right hand in oblique view

Hand Lateral View

Positioning of Patient: The patient is seated with the medial aspect of the forearm resting on the table and the medial aspect of hand and little finger in contact with the film, fingers are extended and the thumb abducted and supported on a non-opaque pad. A sandbag is placed on the forearm for immobilisation.

Direction and Centring of X-ray Beam: The vertical ray is directed to the head of 2nd metacarpal bone.

True lateral view of hand is usually not helpful.

Distance 90 cm KvP 50 mAs 12

Posteroanterior Hand with Ulnar Deviation (PA with Hand Abducted)

Positioning of Patient: The patient is seated at the side or end of the table with arm partly abducted and the pronated forearm resting on the table with anterior aspect of wrist in contact with the cassette; keeping the radial and ulnar styloid process equidistance from the cassette, the hand is adducted and immobilised in this position.

Film size 10" × 8"

Direction and Centring of X-ray Beam: The vertical central ray is directed midway between the radial and ulnar styloid process.

Distance 90 cm KvP 45 mAs 8

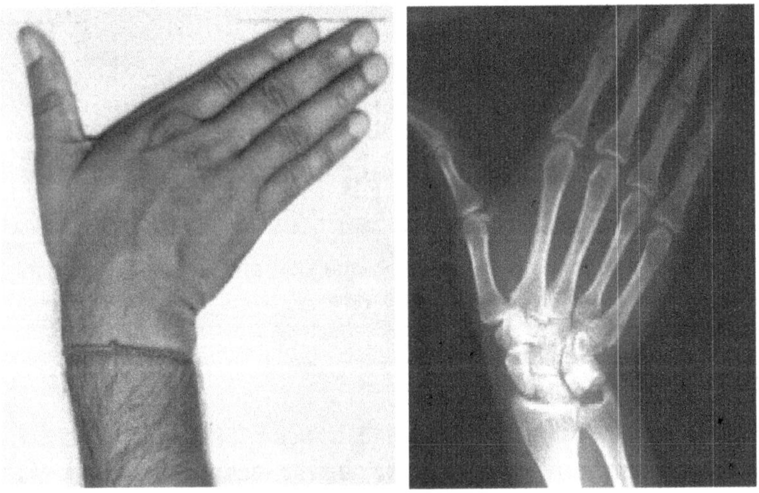

Fig. 2.63: Position of hand in ulnar deviation and X-ray of hand in ulnar deviation

Wrist: Posteroanterior View

Positioning of Patient: Patient is seated at the table with elbow flexed to a right angle and the arm abducted to allow the anterior aspect of forearm and palm to rest on the table. Preferably shoulder, elbow and wrist should be at same horizontal/level. The fingers are slightly flexed to bring the anterior aspect of wrist in close contact with the film and radial and ulnar styloid processes are equidistant from the film.

Direction and Centring of X-ray Beam: The vertical central ray is directed to a point midway between radial and ulnar styloid process.

Film size 10" × 8"

Distance 90 cm KvP 54 mAs 12

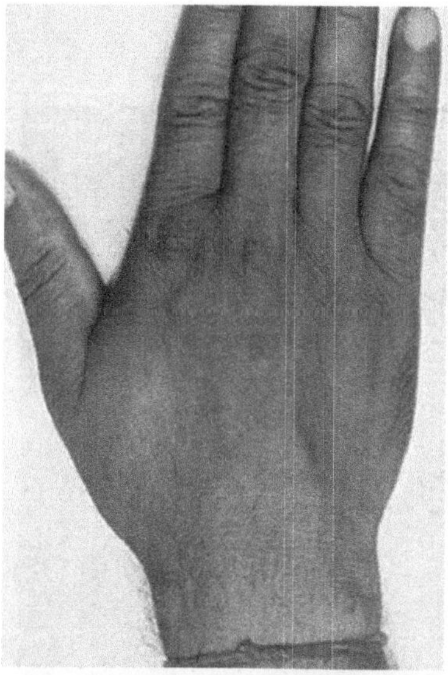

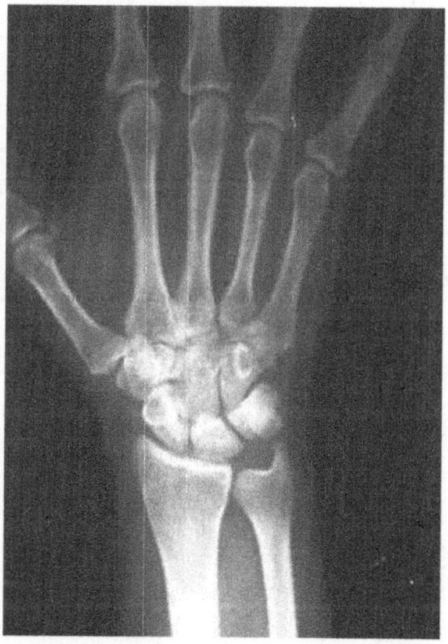

Fig. 2.64: Position of hand for wrist joint PA view and skiagram of wrist joint posteroanterior (PA) view

Wrist: Lateral View

Positioning of Patient: From the position for posteroanterior, the hand is laterally rotated through 90° to bring the palm of the hand at right angle to the table. The film is kept under the wrist. Radial and ulnar styloid processes are superimposed.

Direction and Centring of X-ray Beam: The vertical central ray is directed to the radial styloid process.

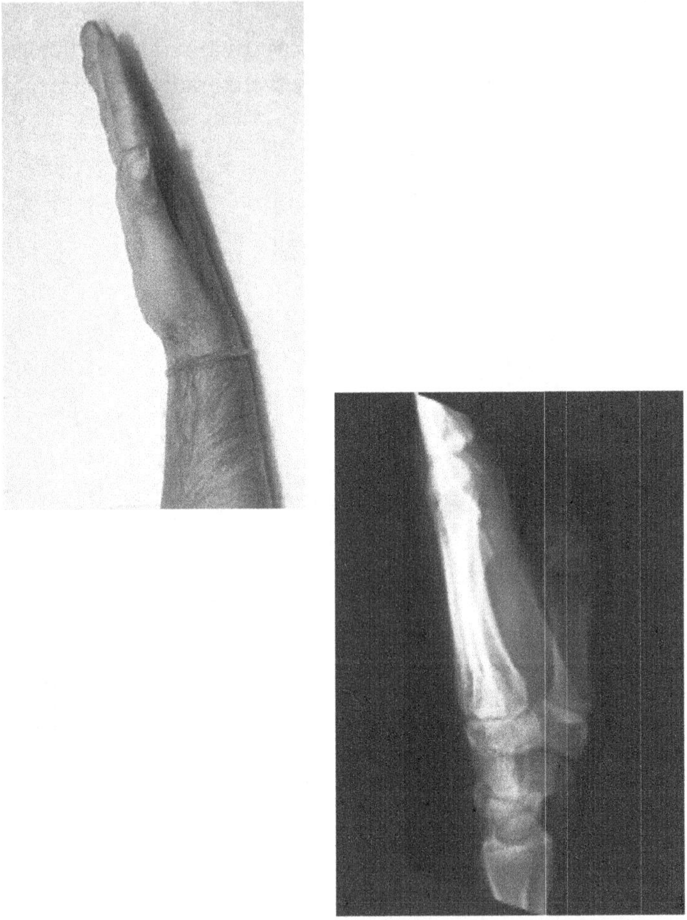

Fig. 2.65: Position of hand for wrist joint lateral view and skiagram of wrist joint lateral view

LOWER EXTREMITY

Femur

Film size 15" × 6" or 14" × 17"

Anteroposterior View: Patient lies supine on table with leg fully extended. The foot is rotated a little inwards medially so that patella is parallel with the table. To restrict the mobility sandbag is placed over the leg.

Direction and Centring of the X-ray Beam: Central rays are aligned over middle of thigh at right angle to the film.

Distance 90 cm KvP 60 mAs 20

Grid No

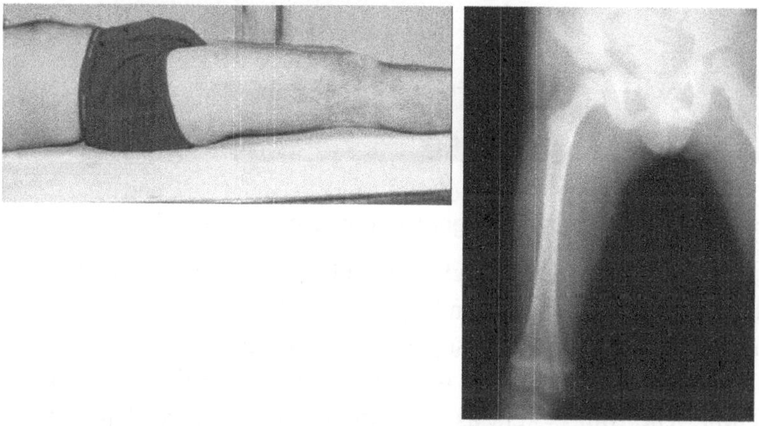

Fig. 2.66: Position for femur AP view and skiagram of right femur in AP view

Lateral View: Patient lying on affected side with tibia and fibula in true lateral position and lateral border of foot on the table. Knee joint should be included and a sandbag is placed over leg to minimize the mobility of the leg.

Direction and Centring of the X-ray Beam: Central rays are aligned over the middle of thigh at right angles to the film.

Exposure factor remains same as in AP view.

Distance 90 cm KvP 56 mAs 20

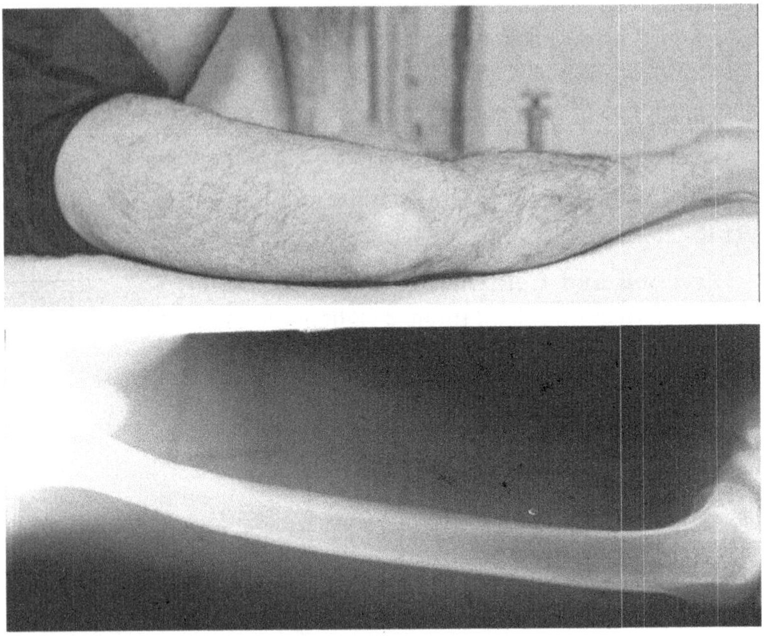

Fig. 2.67: Position of right femur in lateral view and skiagram of right femur in lateral position

View for Intercondylar Notch: This view is useful to demonstrate loose bodies in knee joint and increased size in cases of haemophilia. Patient lies supine. The knee which is to be examined is flexed for 60°. The limb is rotated to centralise the patella over femur. The film is kept as close to posterior aspect of femur as possible using sandbag. The use of curved cassette will better delineate.

Direction and Centring of the X-ray Beam: Centre immediately below the apex of patella with centrally directed at 110° to the axis of tibia to demonstrate anterior part of notch and at 90° to axis of tibia to demonstrate the posterior part of the notch.

Distance 90 cm KvP 66 mAs 30

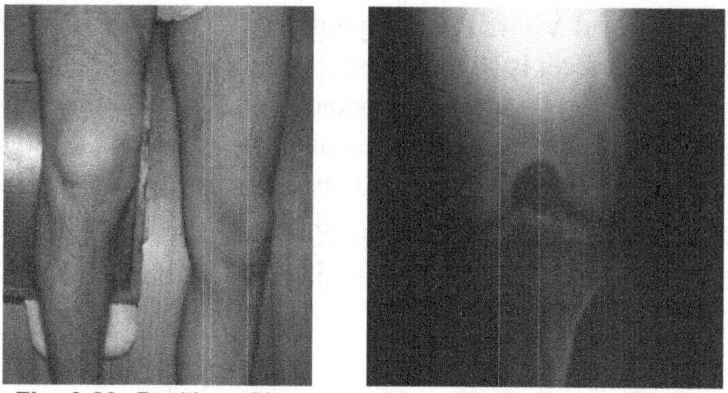

Fig. 2.68: Position of intercondylar notch view and skiagram view of intercondylar notch

Knee Joint

Anteroposterior View: Patient sitting or lying on table, leg fully extended and rotated slightly inwards so that the patella is centralized over the femur. Sandbag is placed over tibia and fibula.

This position can be utilised for single or bilateral knee joint skiagram in AP position.

Direction and Centring of the X-ray Beam: Central rays 1.5 cm below the lower border of patella at right angles to the film (Fig. 2.35).

Film size 10" × 8" for single joint and 12" × 12" for both knee joints.

Distance 90 cm KvP 56 mAs 20

Grid No

(a) (b)

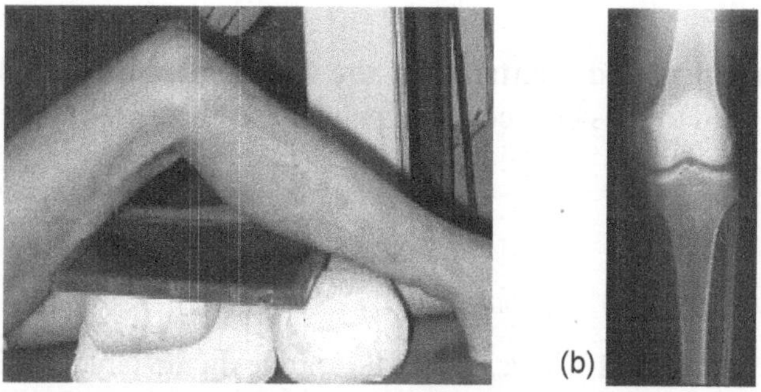

Fig. 2.69: (a) Single or both knee joints AP view (b) X-ray of right knee AP view

Knee Lateral View: Patient lying on affected side with knee slightly flexed. Heel is slightly raised from the table and the knee under examination should be in contact with film. The other leg is brought over the affected one and should be resting on the table in front of it. Knee lateral view is usually taken as single exposure.

Direction and Centring of the X-ray Beam: Central rays is aligned 2.5 cm below and 2.5 cm behind the lower border of patella.

Film size 10" × 8"

Distance 90 cm KvP 56 mAs 16

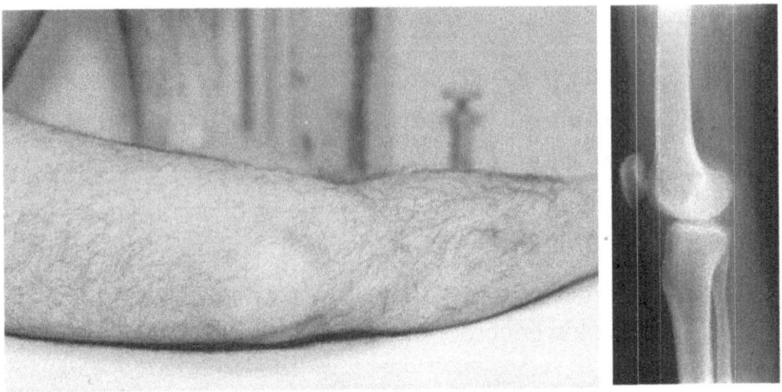

Fig. 2.70: Knee lateral view

Anteroposterior View in Erect Position (Weight Bearing): This is indicated to demonstrate the angle of femur to the tibia in genu valgus, varus like conditions. Ideally both knees are radiographed on one film.

Direction and Centring of the X-ray Beam: Central rays are aligned to pass between both patella at right angles to the film.

Patella

Film size either 10" × 8" or 6½" × 8½"

Skyline/Axial View: Patient lies prone on the table. Tibia and fibula should be steadied either by a bandage or held by hand, in flexed position. Close to back of femur.

Direction and Centring of X-ray Beam: Central rays over patella at an angle of 15° to lower leg cephalad.

Distance 90 cm KvP 60 mAs 24

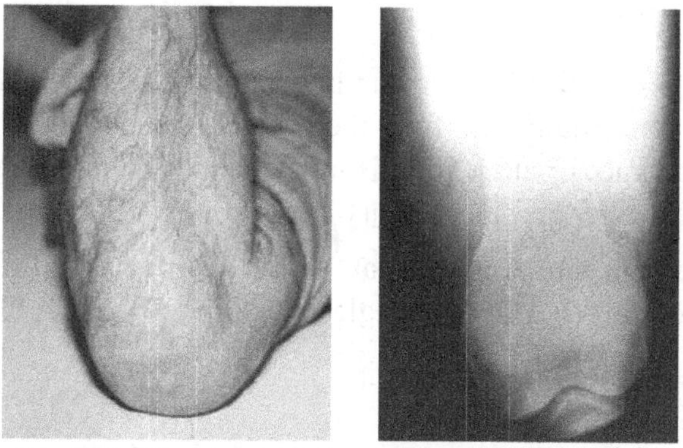

Fig. 2.71: Position of knee in skyline position and X-ray of knee (for patella) in skyline position

Caution: In cases of suspected transverse fracture of patella, this view should not be employed as the fractured segments would be more widely separated.

Modified View: Patient sits with affected knee in flexed position at an angle of 135° and the foot resting on a sandbag. Cassette is supported vertically about 15 cm proximal to femoral condyle.

Direction and Centring of X-ray Beam: Central rays are aligned at the level of foot is directed upward at an angle of 10°. Gonads should be shielded.

Posteroanterior View of Patella: The patient lies prone with a small pad placed under the ankle for comfort. The leg is extended.

Direction and Centring of X-ray Beam: Central rays are aligned over the bend of knee at right angle to the films.

Medial and Lateral Oblique View of Patella: Patient lies prone on table with the extended knee and sandbag is placed under the ankle. Rotate the leg slightly inwards for medial oblique view and slightly outwards for lateral oblique view.

Direction and Centring of X-ray Beam: Central rays are aligned over the bend of knee on medial and lateral side alternatively at right angle to the film.

Leg

Anteroposterior View: Patient lies supine on table with leg fully extended are equidistant from the film. Care should be taken that either the knee or ankle joint is included in film, preferably both. The joint nearer the site of injury must be included in the film.

Direction and Centring of X-ray Beam: Central rays over middle of tibia (leg) at right angle to the film.

Film size 15" × 12" or 15" × 6"

Distance 90 cm KvP 54 mAs 12

Grid No

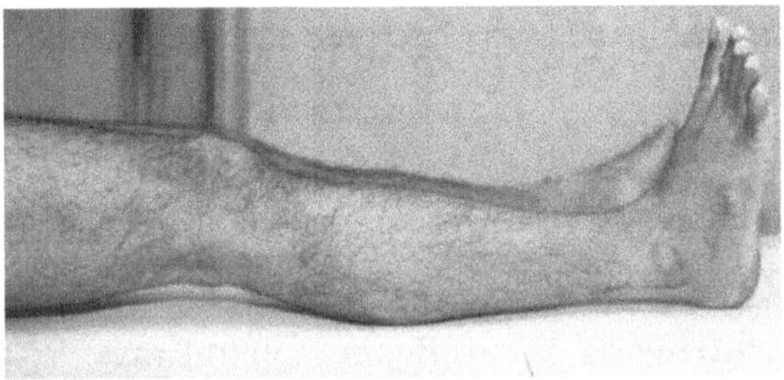

(a)

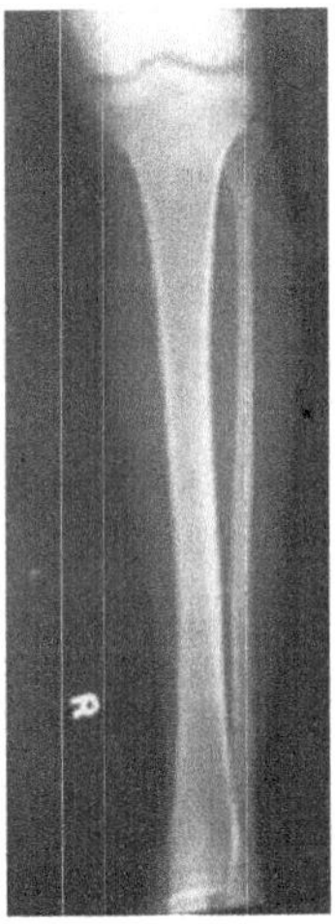

(b)

Fig. 2.72: (a) Position for right leg AP view
(b) X-ray for right leg AP view

Lateral View: Patient lying on affected side, the knee is flexed with lateral border of foot on the table; keeping malleoli superimposed on each other. Unaffected leg is brought over the affected one and rests on table in front of it, sandbag is placed over lower end of femur.

Direction and Centring of X-ray Beam: Central rays over middle of tibia at right angle to the film.

Film size 15" × 12" or 15" × 6"

Distance 90 cm KvP 50 mAs 12

Grid No

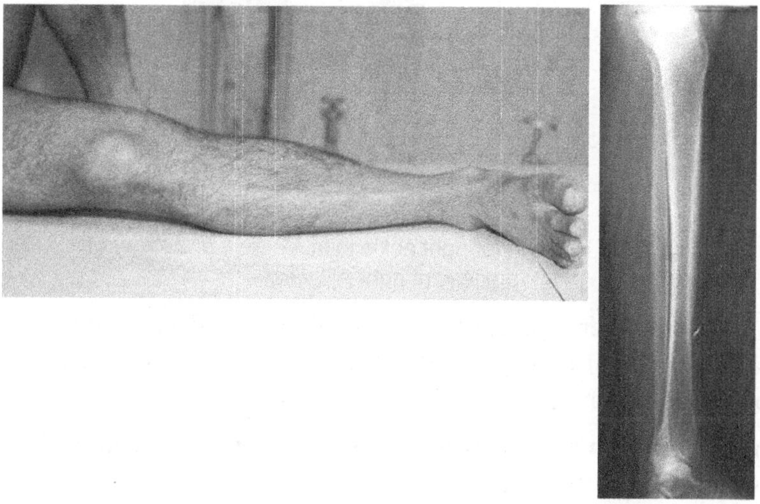

Fig. 2.73: Position for right leg in lateral view and X-ray of right leg in lateral view

Ankle Joint

Anteroposterior View: Patient supine on table with ankle resting on film. The foot should be as near vertical as possible to avoid superimposition of calcaneum over ankle joint. Foot is turned inwards until both the malleoli are equidistant from the film. Sandbag is resting against sole of foot.

Direction and Centring of X-ray Beam: Central rays over midpoint between the malleoli at right angle to the film.

Film size 6½" × 8½"

Distance 90 cm KvP 50 mAs 12

Grid No

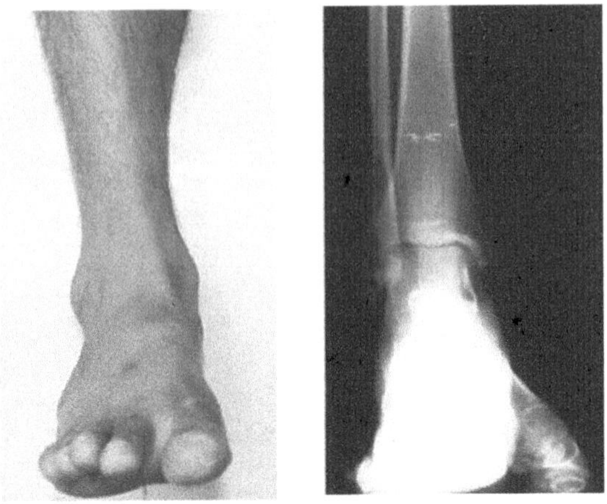

Fig. 2.74: Position for right ankle joint AP view and X-ray of ankle joint right AP view

Lateral View: Patient lies on the injured or effected side with lateral border of foot on the film. Knee is slightly flexed and rests on a sandbag or pad.

Direction and Centring of the X-ray Beam: Central rays over medial malleolus at right angles to the film.

Distance 90 cm KvP 50 mAs 10

Grid No

(a) (b)

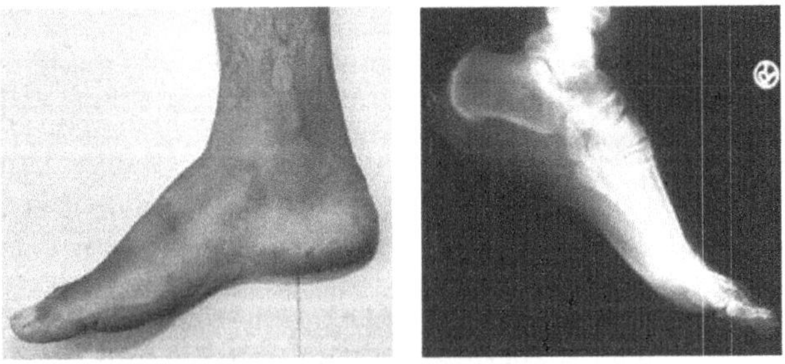

Fig. 2.75: (a) Position for ankle joint lateral view (b) X-ray of ankle joint in lateral view

Anteroposterior in Forced Inversion or Eversion: This is supernumerary view to demonstrate torn medial and lateral ligaments. The patient is positioned for AP view. The ankle is then forcibly inverted or everted by an orthopedic surgeon and held in that position while the exposure is made.

Direction and Centring of the X-ray Beam: Central ray to pass through ankle joint at right angles to the film.

Foot

Anteroposterior (Dorsiplanter) View: Patient supine or seated on table with foot resting flat on film, knee is leaning slightly toward the midline of body.

Direction and Centring of X-ray Beam: Central rays over base of III metatarsal bone at an angle of 15° towards ankle.

Film size 12" × 10" or 10" × 8"

Distance 90 cm KvP 48 mAs 10

Grid No

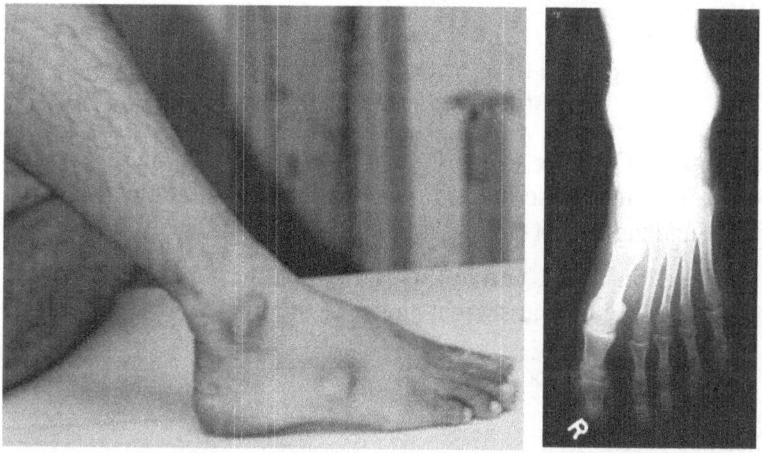

Fig. 2.76: Position for foot AP view and X-ray of right foot AP view

Anteroposterior Oblique (Dorsiplantar Oblique View): From AP position the leg is allowed to lean medially until the sole of the foot is at an angle of 45° to the film. In this position, dorsum of foot is horizontal with the table top.

Direction and Centring of X-ray Beam: Central rays through medial border of foot at the level of navicular with 15° tilts towards ankle.

Film size 12" × 10" or 10" × 8"

Distance 90 cm KvP 52 mAs 12

Grid No

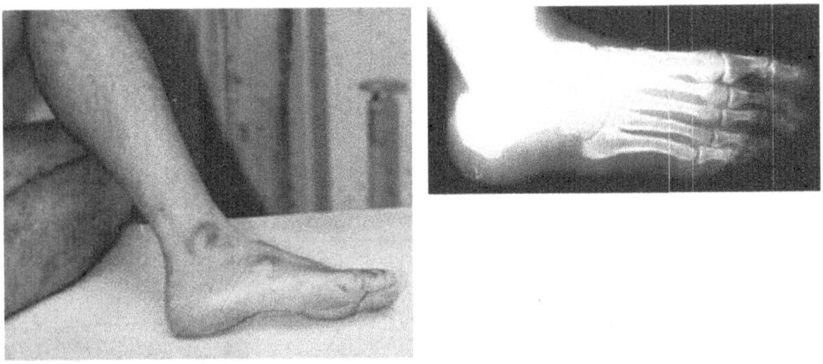

Fig. 2.77: Position for foot AP oblique view and X-ray of foot in AP oblique view

Lateral Oblique View: Patient lies or sits with lateral border of foot on the film so that the sole of foot is at an angle of 45° to film. Sandbag is kept over leg for immobilisation.

Direction and Centring of X-ray Beam: Central rays over base of 5th metatarsal at right angles to the film.

Film size 12" × 10" or 10" × 8"

Distance 90 cm KvP 52 mAs 16

True Lateral View: Patient lies on side with lateral border of foot on the film knee is flexed and resting on a sandbag so that the sole of foot is at right angle to the film.

Direction and Centring of the X-ray Beam: Central rays over middle of foot at right angle to the film.

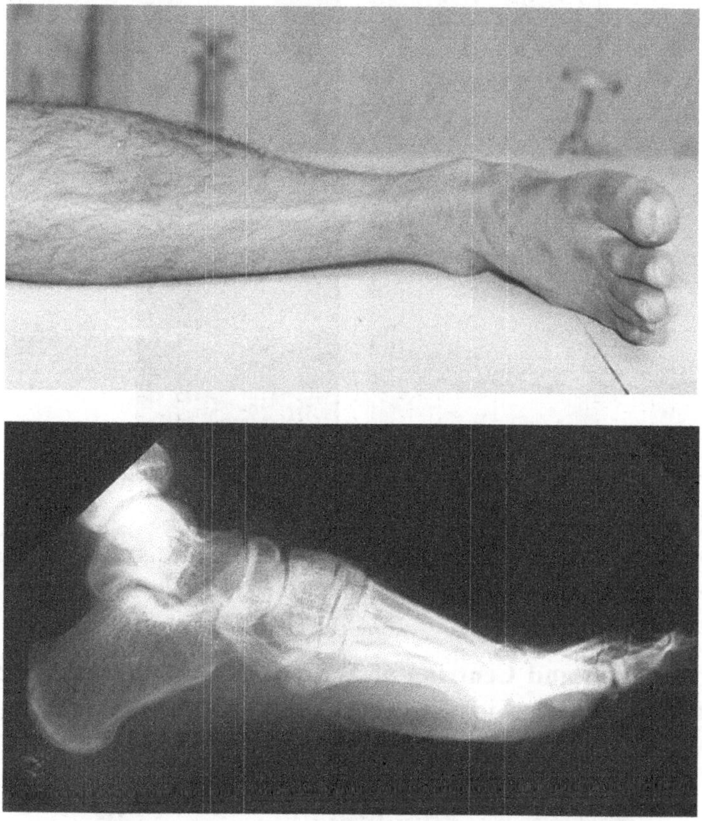

Fig. 2.78: Position for foot lateral view and X-ray foot for lateral view

Toes

Anteroposterior (Dorsiplantar) View: Sole of foot placed flat on film. The toes are separated from each other by pad of cotton wool.

Direction and Centring of the X-ray Beam: Central rays over metatarsophalangeal joint of 3rd toe, at right angles to the film.

Film size 10" × 8"

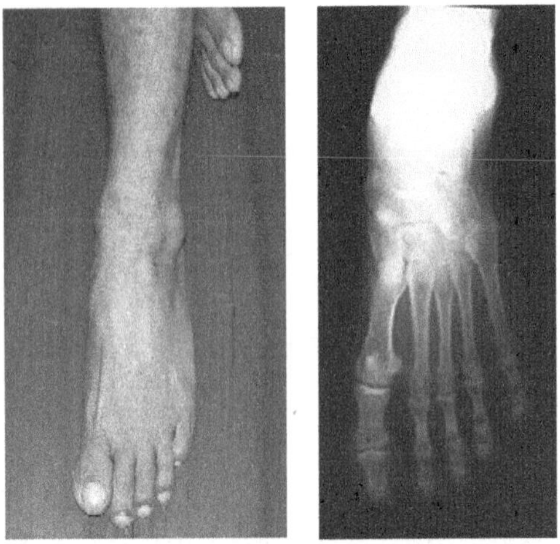

Fig. 2.79: Position for toe anteroposterior view and X-ray for toe AP view

Lateral Oblique View: Patient lies on side or sits on table with lateral border of foot on table. Sole of foot should be at an angle of 45° to the film.

Direction and Centring of X-ray Beam: Central rays over metatarsophalangeal joint of 3rd toe at right angle to the film.

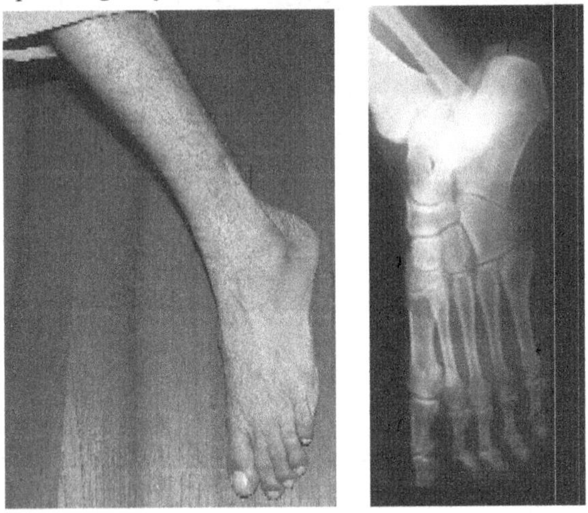

Fig. 2.80: Toe lateral oblique view

True Lateral: For 1st, 2nd, 3rd toe—Foot is placed on its side with medial aspect in contact with film, 4th and 5th toes are held out of way by a cotton bandage.

For 4th and 5th toe, the foot is placed on its side with its lateral aspect in contact with the film. 1st, 2nd, 3rd toes are held out of way by a cotton bandage.

True lateral view of foot is of not useful because of superimposition.

Direction and Centring of X-ray Beam: Central rays over middle phalanx of toe to be radiographed at right angles to the film.

Distance 90 cm KvP 50 mAs 6-8

Grid No

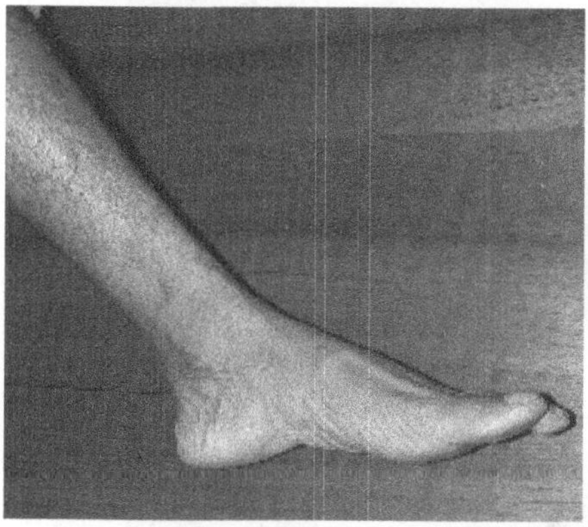

(a)

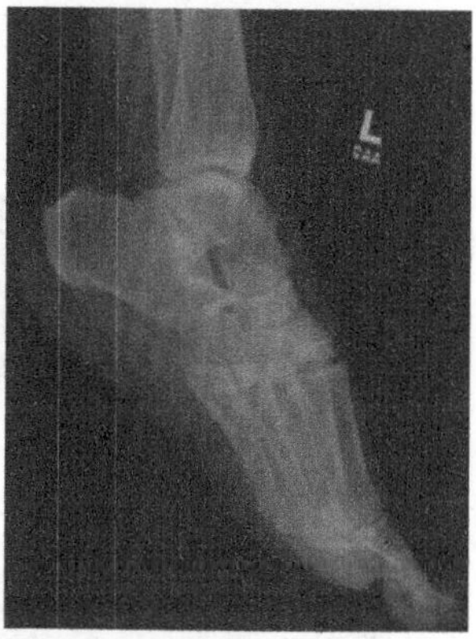

(b)

Fig. 2.81: (a) Position for lateral view foot
(b) X-ray for foot in lateral view

Calcaneum

Lateral View: Patient sits or lies on table with lateral border of foot in contact with the film. Knee is partially flexed with a sandbag under the flexed knee.

Direction and Centring of X-ray Beam: Central rays 2.5 cm below and 2.5 cm behind the medial malleolus.

Film size 6½" × 8½"

Distance 90 cm KvP 55 mAs 8-10

Grid No

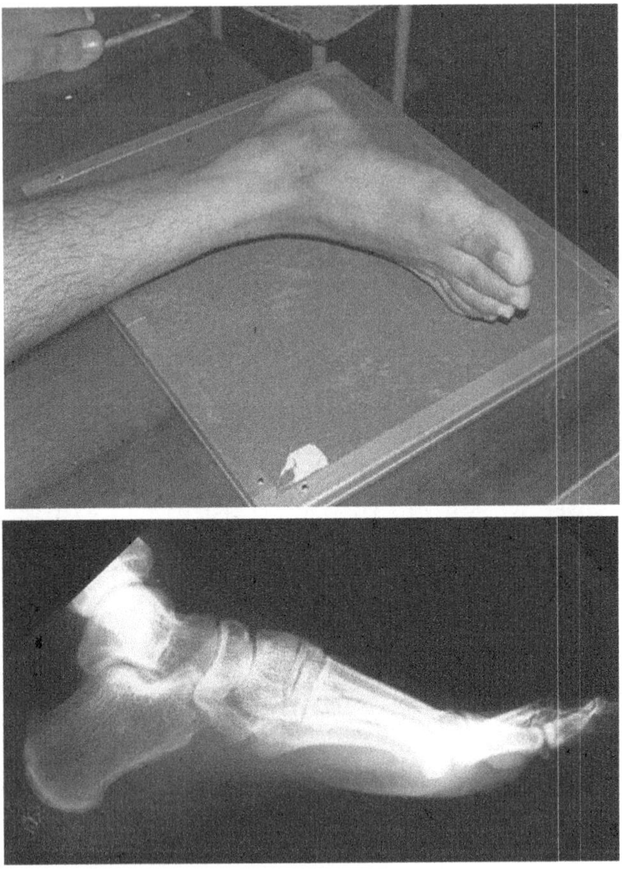

Fig. 2.82: Position for lateral view of calcaneum and X-ray in lateral view of calcaneum

Axial View

Inferosuperior: Patient sitting on table with legs extended and ankle in AP position. The foot is dorsiflexed. A cotton bandage is passed around the foot and held by the patient with both hands to maintain dorsiflexion.

Direction and Centring X-ray Beam: Central rays are aligned to heel with 30° tube angled cephalad.

OR

Superoinferior: Patient stands with heel or heels being examined on the film. Patient bends his knees slightly and leans forward with a chair in front of him for support.

Direction and Centring of X-ray Beam: Central rays over heel or midway between the heels if both are being examined at an angle of 15-20° towards the toes.

Distance 90 cm KvP 60 mAs 20

Grid No

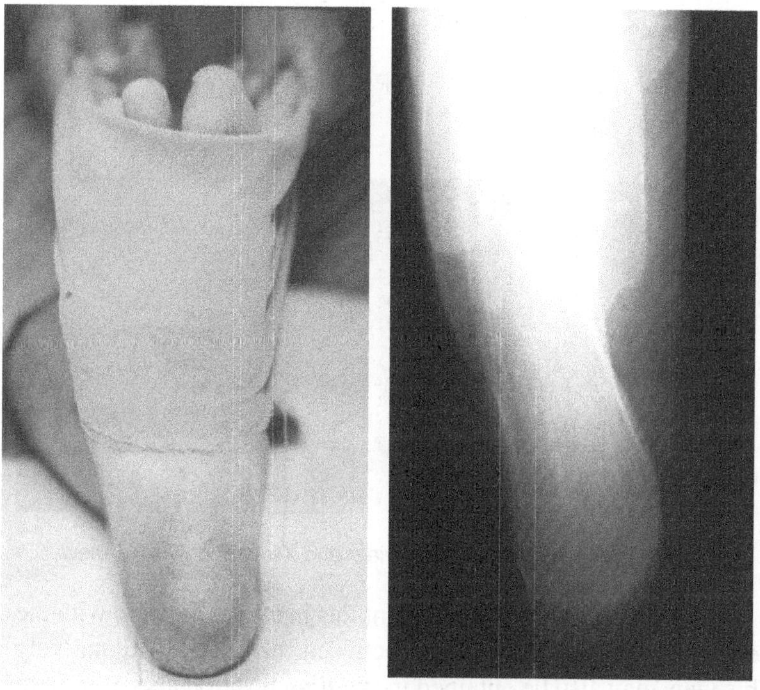

Fig. 2.83: Position for axial view of calcaneum and X-ray of calcaneum in axial view

PELVIS

Pelvis or Pelvic Girdle

Pelvis Anteroposterior View: Patient lying supine on the table with extended legs. The heels are slightly separated with big toes touching each other. The pelvis must be positioned symmetrically with anterior superior iliac spines equidistant from the film.

Direction and Centring of X-ray Beam: Central rays are aligned 2" below the mid point of a line joining anterior superior iliac spine at right angle to the film.

Film size 15" × 12" or 14" × 17" in adults

12" × 10" in children

Distance 90 cm KvP 80 mAs 100

Grid Yes

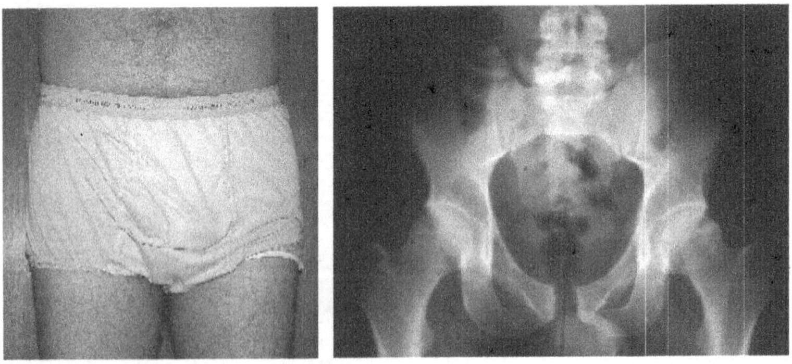

Fig. 2.84: Position of pelvis AP view and X-ray of pelvis AP view

Lateral View of Pelvis: Patient lies in lateral position with the legs extended and a small pad between the knees. Alternatively this view may also be obtained in standing position also. Centre to the upper border of femoral head.

Distance 90 cm KvP 86 mAs 120

Grid Yes

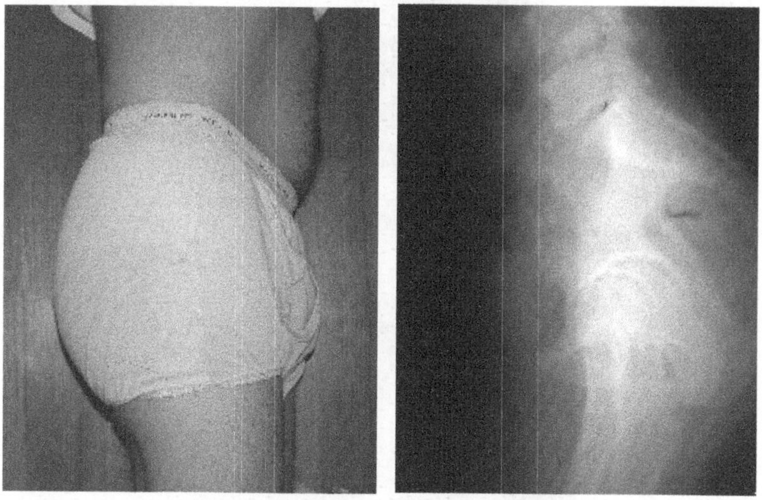

Fig. 2.85: Position of pelvis lateral view

Hip Joint

Anteroposterior View: Patient lies supine on table, leg extended and the foot slightly rotated inwards so that both the malleoli are equidistant from the film. Sandbag is placed over leg for the purpose of immobilisation.

Direction and Centring of X-ray Beam: Central rays are allowed to pass 1" below mid point of a line joining anterior superior iliac spine and upper border of pubic at right angles to the film.

Film size 12" × 10" or according to patient's body built.

Distance 90 cm KvP 72 mAs 60

Grid Yes

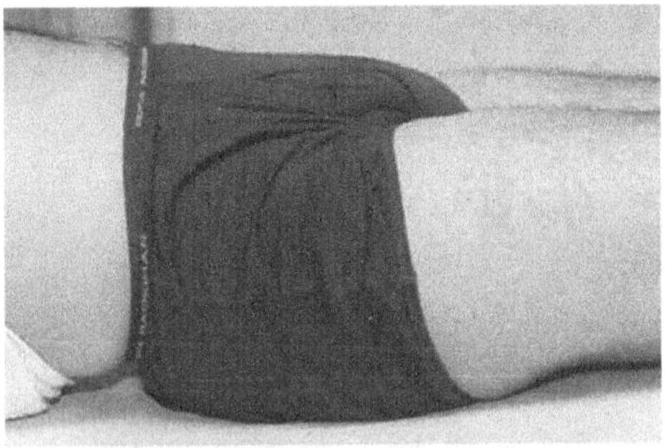

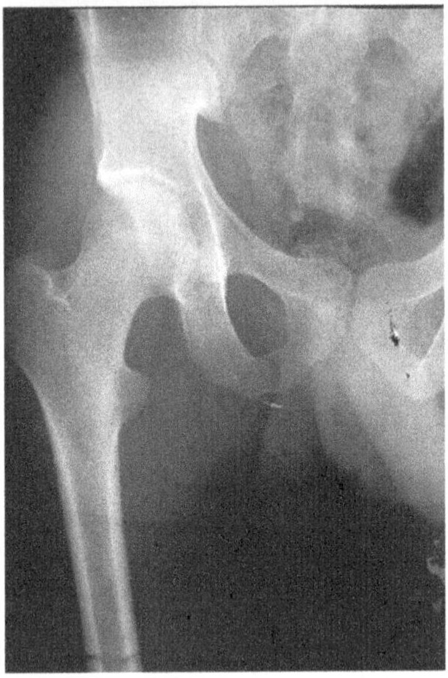

Fig. 2.86: Position of right hip joint AP view and X-ray of right hip joint view

Lateral View of Hip Joint: The patient lies supine with the pelvis raised on foam pads and the injured limb extended, the foot is slightly rotated medially, if possible, to avoid foreshortening of femoral neck. The normal knee is flexed and the foot is placed on a stool out of the way of beam. The film and grid are positioned vertically against the injured hip and adjusted so that the film is parallel with neck of femur.

Film size 12" × 10" or according to patient's body built.

Distance 90 cm KvP 72 mAs 60

Grid Yes

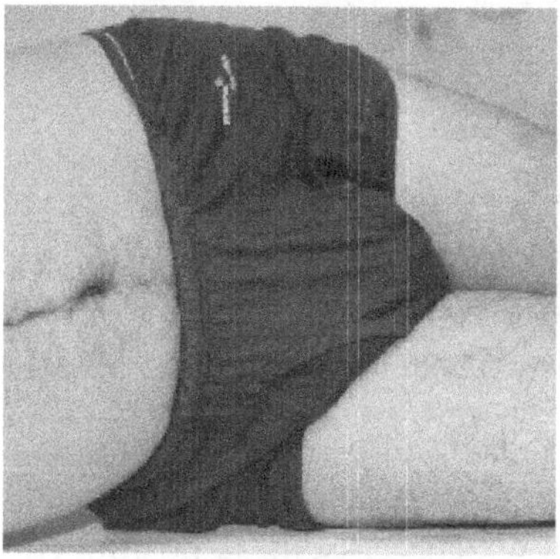

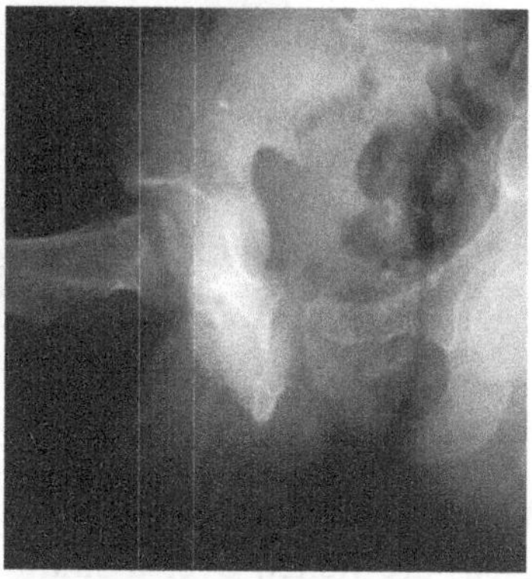

Fig. 2.87: Position for lateral view of hip joint and radiograph showing hip joint lateral view

"Frog Position", Lateral View Both Hips: From AP position draw the patient's knees up until the feet are flat on the table. Then rotate the legs outwards as far as possible (45°-60°) resting the soles of the feet together. The thighs should be resting symmetrically on equal sized foam pads.

Direction and Centring of X-ray Beam: Central rays are aligned 1" (2.5 cm) above the pubic symphysis at right angle to the film.

Film size 15" × 12"

Distance 90 cm KvP 72 mAs 60

Grid Yes

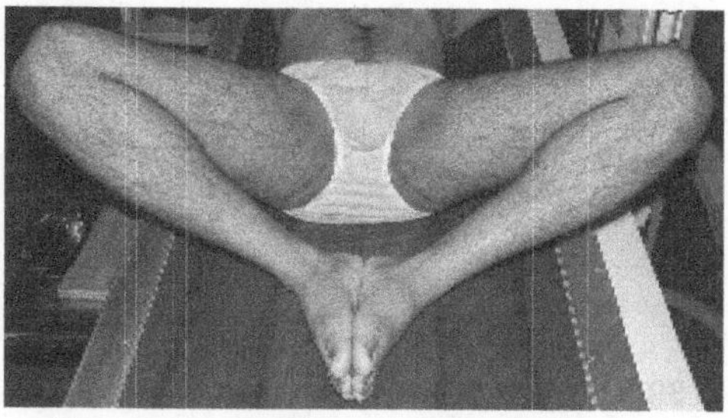

Fig. 2.88a: Patient's position for frog view

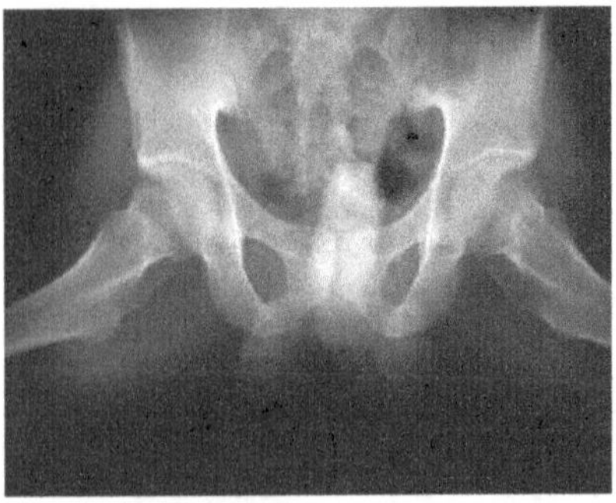

Fig. 2.88b: Frog position of both hip joints

Sacrum

Anteroposterior (AP) View: Patient lies supine on the table and knees are flexed over a small pillow. The cassette is positioned such that its upper border is at the level of iliac crest.

Direction and Centring of X-ray Beam: Centre at 2" (5 cm) above the symphysis pubis in midline with rays directed 15° cephalad.

Film size 12" × 10" or according to patient's body built.

Distance 90 cm KvP 80 mAs 100

Grid Yes

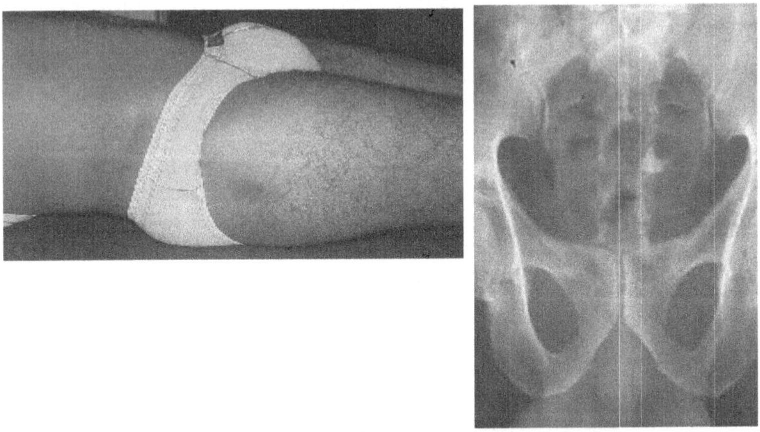

Fig. 2.89: Position of patient for sacral vertebrae and skiagram of sacrum AP view

Lateral View: The patient is rotated in true lateral position so that the sacrum is approximately over the centre of the table. Cotton pad is kept under mid lumbar region to straighten the vertebral column. The knees are flexed.

Direction and Centring of X-ray Beam: Centring made at a highest point of pelvis in lateral position.

Film size 12" × 10" or according to patient's body built.

Distance 90 cm KvP 86 mAs 160

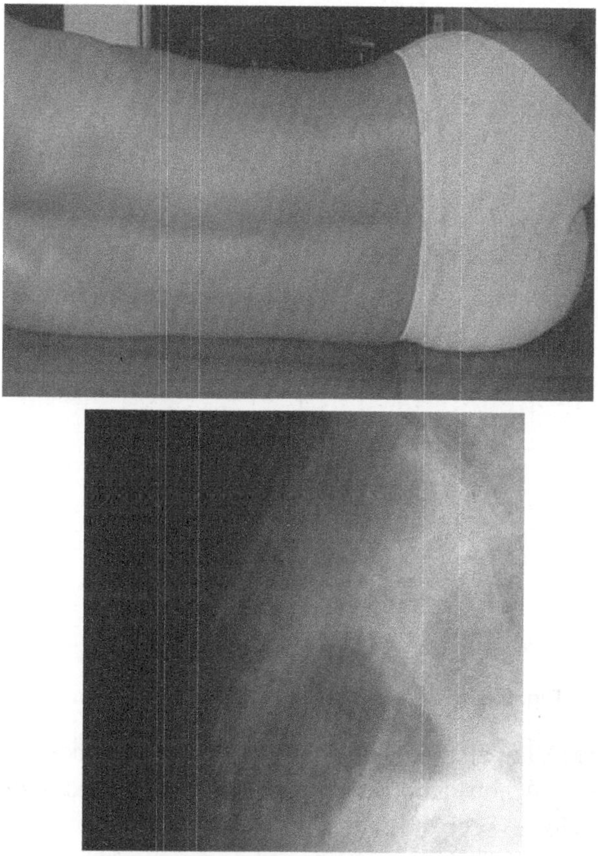

Fig. 2.90: Position of patient for lateral view of sacrum and skiagram of lateral view of sacrum

Coccyx

Anteroposterior View: Patient lies supine on the table with both knee flexed and supported by sandbag.

Direction and Centring of X-ray Beam: Central rays are aligned over midline of body at the level of upper of symphysis pubis at an angle of 10-15° toward the feet.

Film size 12" × 10" or according to patient's body built.

Distance 90 cm KvP 80 mAs 160

Grid Yes

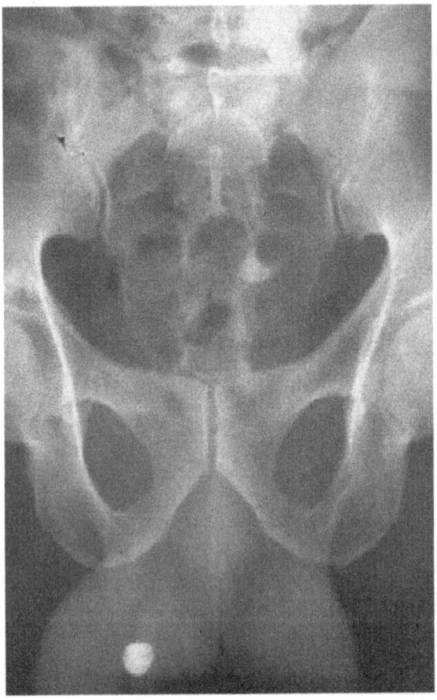

Fig. 2.91: Position of patient for coccyx AP view

Lateral View: Patient lying on side in true lateral position with flexed knee. A non radioopaque pad should be placed under mid lumbar region to keep the patient in position.

Direction and Centring of X-ray Beam: Central ray at the level of upper border of symphysis pubis over the patient's buttocks at right angles to the film.

Film size 12" × 10" or according to patient's body built.

Distance 90 cm KvP 90 mAs 200

Grid Yes

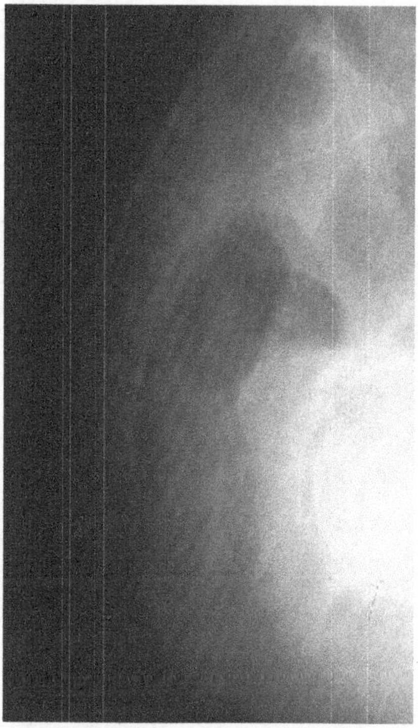

Fig. 2.92: Position of patient for coccyx lateral view see Figure 2.90 and skiagram showing lateral view of coccyx

Sacroiliac Joint

Anteroposterior View: Patient lies supine on table with knees touching each other and slightly flexed. Pelvis should be positioned symmetrically.

Direction and Centring of the X-ray Beam: Central rays are aligned 5 cm above pubic symphysis in midline at an angle of 15° cephalad.

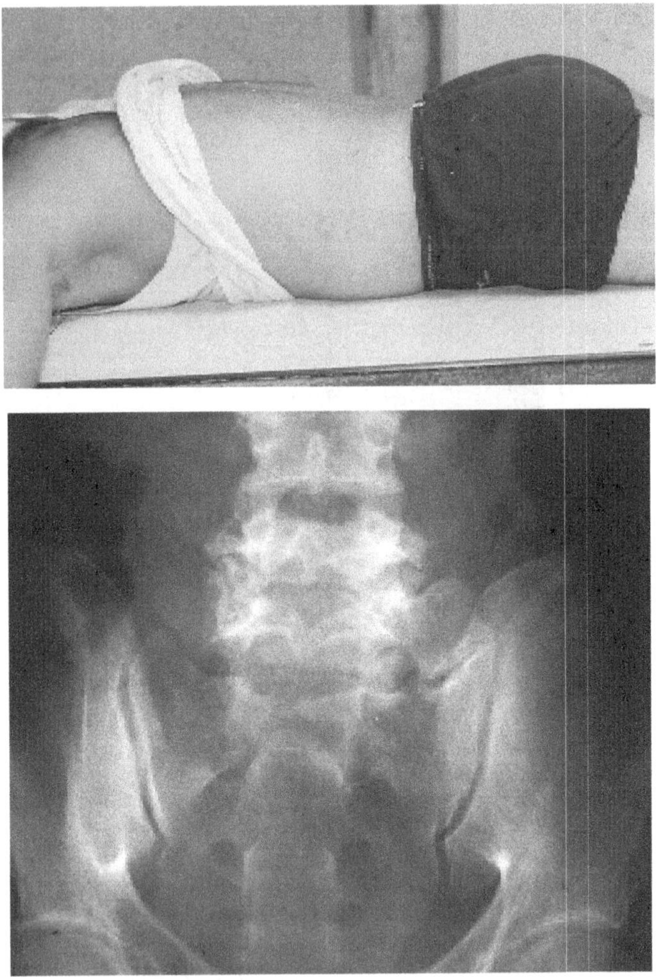

Fig. 2.93: Position of patient for AP view SI joint and Skiagram sacroiliac joint AP view

Posteroanterior (PA) View: Patient lies prone on table with symmetrical pelvis.

Direction and Centring of X-ray Beam: Central rays are aligned in midline to the mid sacral region with ray directed 15° cephalad.

Distance 90 cm KvP 80 mAs 100

Grid Yes

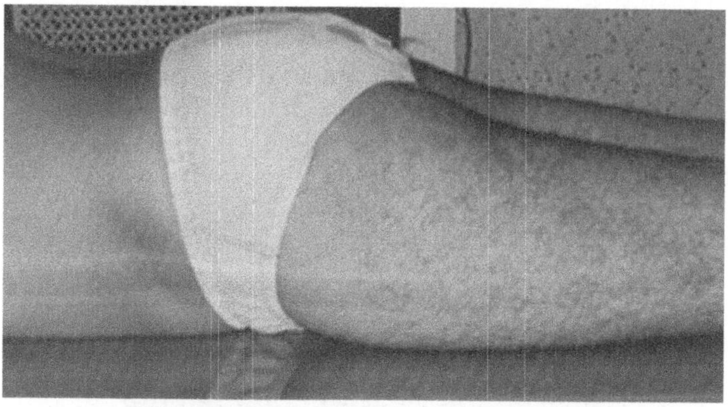

Fig. 2.94a: Position of patient for PA view of SI joint

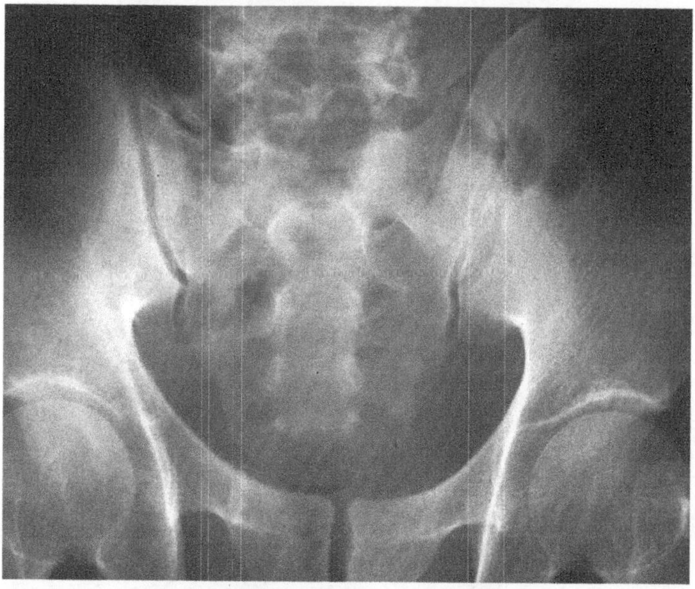

Fig. 2.94b: Skiagram for SI joint PA view

Oblique Views: Both oblique views should be taken for comparison from supine position, the patient is rotated 20-25° to either side in turn. The knee nearer the table is flexed and the pelvis is supported by sandbag.

Direction and Centring of X-ray Beam: Centre at 1-1.5" medial to the anterior superior iliac spine on the raised side with ray perpendicular to the film.

Distance 90 cm KvP 80 mAs 100

Grid Yes

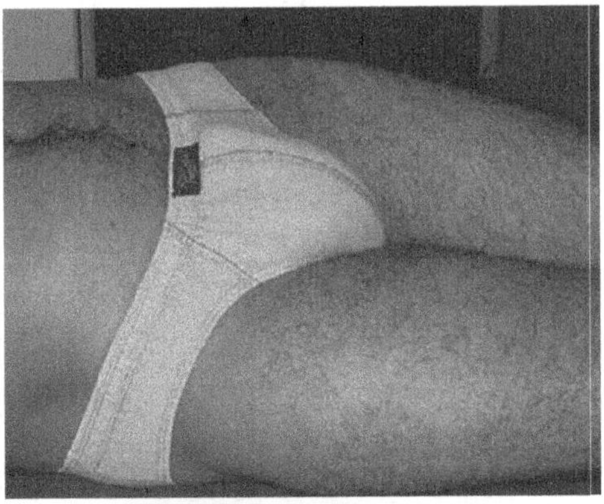

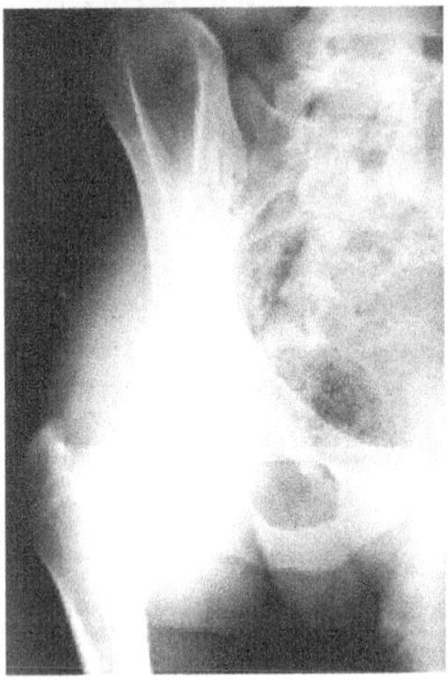

Fig. 2.95: Position of patient for Rt./Lt. oblique view of SI joint and skiagram showing SI joint oblique view

3

Radiological Procedures Including Contrast Media

GENERAL CONSIDERATIONS

Radiological investigations are indicated in all the systems of human body except for hair and skin. Contraindications are relative or absolute, the factors that increases the risk to the patient can be considered under 3 headings:

Due to Radiation

Except for USG and MRI, all other investigation involves the use of ionizing radiation which are harmful to all tissues especially the developing fetus. In females, 10-day rule (10 days after LMP) must be followed.

The patients exempted from this rule are:

1. Females who deny recent sexual act.
2. Females who are menstruating at the time.
3. Females who have been taking oral contraceptive pills for not less than 3 months.
4. Females who have an IUCD for not less than 3 months.
5. Females who have had undergone sterilization operation.

Irradiation of a fetus during first few weeks of gestation will induce a spontaneous abortion.[(Unscear 1972)] Risks of inducing malignancies or malformations may result from irradiation in later stages of pregnancy.[(Otake and Schull 1984)] The risk of malformation is greatest when the fetus is irradiated during the period of organogenesis (4-8 weeks).

Clinicians and radiologists should consider all female from pregnancy point of view if her menstrual cycle is overdue or missed unless she is definitely known not to be pregnant. To rule out, a pregnancy test may be helpful. However, if at all the pregnant female needs to go for a radiological investigations then her abdomen and pelvis should be protected from radiation by using protective shields.

Due to Contrast Medium

Generalised contraindications to an intravascular contrast medium are as follows:

1. Sensitivity to iodine (iodism).
2. Previous severe adverse reaction—This carries a 30% risk of a similar reaction on a subsequent occasion. The risk is lowered if low osmolar contrast media are used.
3. Heart disease—Cardiac failure and arrhythmias can be precipitated due to sodium-overload.
4. Hepatic failure.
5. Oliguric renal failure.
6. Thyrotoxicosis.
7. Pregnancy.

Due to Technique

Skin sepsis may occur at the needle puncture site.

Patient's Preparation

1. Will admission to hospital be necessary?
2. Any female presenting for radiography at a time when her period is known to be overdue should be considered to be pregnant unless there is information indicating the absence of pregnancy.

If her cycle is so irregular that it is difficult to know whether a period has been missed, then a pregnancy test or pelvic USG examination may help to determine whether she is pregnant.

3. The procedure should be explained to the patient and consent should be obtained when necessary.
4. Bowel preparation:
   a. Prior to investigation of GIT.
   b. When considerable faecal loading obscures other intra-abdominal organs.
   c. When opacification of an organ is likely to be poor, i.e., the gallbladder in oral cholecystography.

   For other radiological investigations of abdominal organs, bowel preparation is not always necessary and when given, may result in excessive bowel gas. Bowel gas is reduced if the patient is ambulant for 2 hours prior to the examination and those who routinely take laxatives should continue to do so.(Payne-Jeremiah 1977)
5. Previous films and notes should be obtained.
6. The area to be punctured should be cleaned and shaved properly.
7. Pre-medication is necessary for painful procedures. Suggested pre-medication for adult are:
   a. Diazepam 10 mg I.M.
   b. Papaveretum 10 mg I.M.
   c. Useful drugs for children are:
      - Promethazine

        6-12 months—10 mg

        1-5 years—15-20 mg

        5-10 years—20-25 mg
      - Trimeprazine—4 mg/kg
      - Brandy—5-20 ml.
8. The patient should micturate (Pass urine) if advised prior to the procedure.

Preliminary Films

Purpose

1. To make any final adjustments in exposure factors, centring, collimation and patient's position for which the film should always be taken using the same equipment as will be used to the remainder of the position.
2. To exclude prohibitive factors such as residual from a previous examination or overlying faeces.
3. To demonstrate, identify and localize opacities which may be obscured by contrast medium.
4. To elicit radiological physical signs.

The films should have the patient's name, registration no., date and side marker (right or left). The examination can only be proceeded if satisfactory preliminary films have been obtained.

Technique

1. For aseptic technique the skin is cleaned with chlorhexidine 0.5% in 70% spirit or equivalent.
2. Local anesthetic used is lignocaine 1% **without** adrenaline.
3. Gonad protection is used whenever possible, unless it obscures the region of interest.

Films: When films are taken during the procedure rather than at the end of it, they have for convenience been described under techniques.

After care: May be considered as:

1. Instructions to the patient.
2. Instructions to the ward.

Complications: May be considered under three headings.

Due to Anaesthetic

- General anesthesia.
- Local anesthesia
  - i. Allergic
  - ii. Toxic.

Symptoms are of paresthesia and trembling which may progress to convulsions, cardiovascular and respiratory depression and death.

Due to Contrast Media

Incidence is highest in the very young and very old patient but there is no sex difference.

Adverse Reaction: Incidence 5%.

Classified into:

1. Major reaction—i.e., those that interfere with the examination and require treatment.
2. Minor reaction—Those that interfere with the examination but do not require treatment.
3. Trivial reaction—Those that do not interfere with examination and require only firm reassurance.

Prophylaxis for Adverse Reaction:

1. Pre-testing.
2. Pre-treatment with steroid.
3. Pre-treatment with anti-histamine.
4. Change of contrast medium to a low-osmolar contrast medium.
5. Reduction of patient anxiety and apprehention.(Lalli 1980)

Due to Technique

i. Local.
ii. Distant or generalized.

The absorption of X-ray by the tissue of the body and thus their radiographic density depends on the atomic weight of principle substance of which the tissue are composed with. The exception of bone and certain calcified structure that contain Ca and other radio-paque salts. Most of the tissue are composed of C, H and O_2 which have low atomic weight and display very small difference in density. Bone is denser than the other tissue.

The details of certain fine structure of the organ lacks behind in contrast. Artificial method of delineating of such organs are required and so a suitable contrast medium is employed.

The contrast medium may have either a high atomic weight and provide +ve contrast or a low atomic weight and provide –ve contrast. For example of +ve contrast are $BaSO_4$ and organic iodine compound. For example –ve contrast media are gases such as air, CO_2 and O_2.

The selection of the appropriate contrast medium is governed by five important factors:

1. It must be non-toxic.

   Toxic–means poisonous. The term is also used to describe an illness, i.e., caused by poisonous substance.
2. It must produce adequate contrast (not too less contrast medium or too more contrast) so that in small quantity the contrast covers it.
3. It must have a suitable viscosity.
4. It must have a suitable persistence.

   (Some contrast medium remain in the body for several years.)
5. It must be miscibility or immiscibility.

   (It mix with contrast of a structure or it remain in a bolus form and does not mix.)

INTRAVASCULAR CONTRAST MEDIA

The first reports of opacification of the urinary tract by renal excretion rather than by retrograde introduction of a contrast agent appeared in 1923 with the use of 10% sodium iodide. This was followed by iodine derivatives of pyridine, e.g., Uroselectan and diodone (Diodrast) which were utilized in urography from the 1930s.

It was not until 1950 that the modern water-soluble contrast media were introduced into clinical radiology. These are all derivatives of triiodo benzoic acid, the first being sodium acetrizoate.

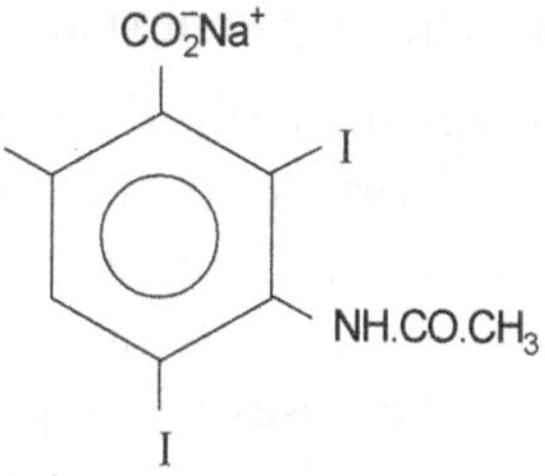

In 1955 a much safer derivative was reported—diatrizoate. This had an acetamido group at the previously unsubstituted position 5 and unlike acetrizoate was fully saturated benzoic acid derivative. Isomerization of diatrizoate and substitution at position 5 of N-methyl carbamyl produced the iothalamate molecule in 1962. The majority of modern conventional water-soluble contrast media are distinguished by differences at position 5 of the anion and by the cations sodium and meglumine.

All conventional ionic water-soluble contrast media are hypertonic with osmolalities of 1200-2000 mosmol kg^{-1} water, 4-7 × the osmolality of blood. Hyperosmolarity is responsible for many of the adverse effects of contrast media and it was primarily to reduce these side-effects that the low osmolar contrast media were developed.

In order to decrease the osmolality without changing the iodine concentration the ratio between the number of iodine atoms and the number of dissolved particles must be increased.

In 1972, a new agent was introduced for radiculography. This was produced by linking two iothalamate molecules to form a dimmer—iocarmate (Dimer X).

Further development has proceeded along two separate pathways. The first was again to combine two tri-iodinated benzene rings to produce an anion with six iodine atoms. Replacement of one of the carboxylic acid groups with a non-ionizing radical means that only one cation is necessary for each molecule. This anion, ioxaglate, is marketed as a mixed sodium and meglumine salt. The alternative approach was to produce a compound that does not ionize in solution and so does not provide radiologically useless cations. Contrast media of this type include metrizamide (Amipaque), iopamidol (Niopam) and iohexol (Omnipaque).

For both types of contrast media the ratio of iodine atoms in the molecule to the number of particles in solution is 3:1. Compared with conventional ionic contrast media, the new low-osmolar contrast media show a theoretical halving of osmolarity for equi-iodine solutions. However, because of aggregation of molecules in solution the measured reduction is approximately one-third.

It should be noted that the terms 'low-osmolar' and 'non-ionic' are not synonymous. Metrizamide, iopamidol, iohexol and ioxaglate are all low osmolar but only the first three compounds are also non-ionic. However, there is no clinical difference between ionic and non-ionic low-osmolar contrast media for intravascular use (Ionic contrast media should not be used intrathecally).

Adverse Effects of Contrast Media

These can be classified as:

1. **Immediate anaphylactic or allergic response due to immunological sensitivity:**
   a. Allergic reactions, which include urticaria, conjunctivitis, rhinitis, bronchospasm and angioneurotic oedema.
   b. Acute anaphylaxis, which occurs in a previously sensitized individual within minutes of administering a contrast medium. It is manifested by bronchospasm, glottic oedema, circulatory collapse, abdominal cramps and diarrhoea. The patient may die unless immediate resuscitative steps are taken.
   c. Anaphylactoid reaction, which is as in (b) but occurs in a non-sensitized individual.
2. **Chemotoxic effects:** The anions are probably not a major cause of contrast medium reactions but the cations are clinically toxic. Sodium cations are more toxic than meglumine to brain

and myocardium. Changes in red blood cell morphology are also a direct chemotoxic effect of contrast media.

3. **Hyperosmolar effects:**
   a. Haemodynamic
   b. Cardiac
   c. Endothelial
   d. Red blood cells
   e. Blood-brain barrier.
4. **Anxiety**

Mechanism of Immediate Anaphylactic or Allergic Responses

1. Anaphylaxis not requiring the complement system. The contrast medium molecule acts as an antigen which reacts with a specific mast cell or basophil-fixed IgE or IgG contrast medium antibody or cross-reacts with other antibodies. This interaction causes the expulsion of mast cell granules and the release of histamine, serotonin, heparin, SRS-A kallikrein, kinin and prostaglandins.
2. Anaphylaxis requires the complement system. The pharmacologically active mediators or adverse reactions can be direct immunological activation of the complement system.
   (See Figure 3.1 on the next page)
3. Direct effect on mast cells. Contrast media have a direct effect on mast cells, basophils and platelets to release histamine. Meglumine salts have the greatest ability to do this and bronchospasm is 4 times more frequent following administration of meglumine salts compared with sodium salts.

Conventional Versus Low-osmolar Contrast Media

Acute Toxicity:

New low-osmolar contrast media have less toxicity than conventional contrast media.

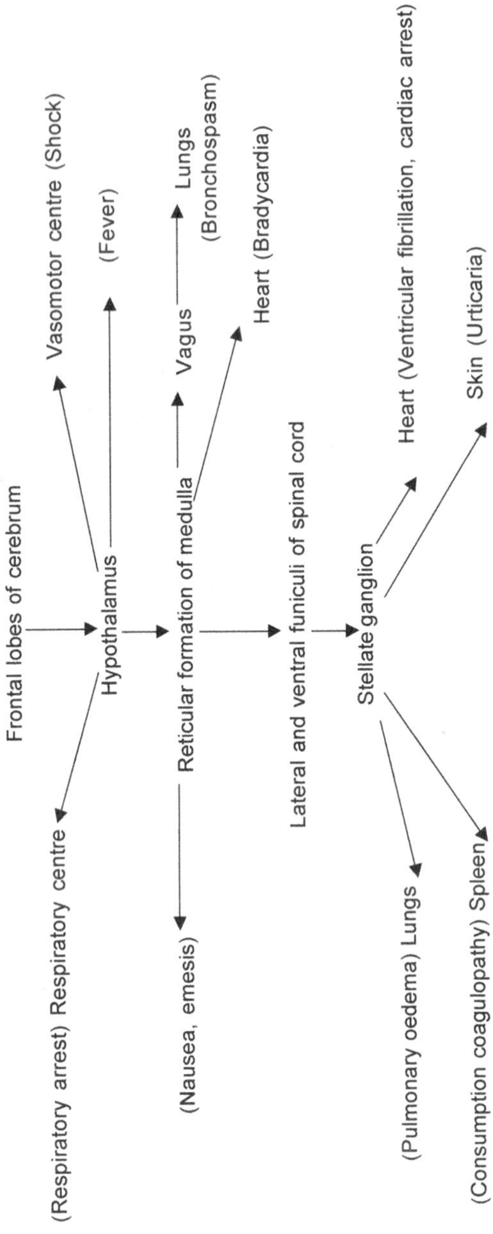

Fig. 3.1: Central nervous system and contrast media reactions

Haemodynamic and Systemic Effects:

The injection of a hypertonic contrast medium causes significant fluid and ion shifts. Immediately after injection there is a significant increase in serum osmolarity. This causes an influx of water from the interstitial space into the vascular compartment, an increase in blood volume and an increase in cardiac output. These effects are particularly important in young children and those with cardiac impairment.

Injection of a conventional contrast medium produces a significant, transient decrease in systemic arterial pressure, a decrease in peripheral vascular resistance, peripheral vasodilatation, tachycardia and an increase in pulmonary arterial pressure. This is accompanied by perception of heat and with intra-arterial pressure. This is accompanied by perception of heat and with intra-arterial injection there is often pain. Low-osmolar contrast media produce significantly less fluid shifts, change in measurable parameters, heat and pain.

Cardiac Effects:

Coronary arteriography with hypertonic contrast media has adverse inotropic and chronotropic effects on the heart. There is a decrease in peak left ventricular systolic pressure, an increase in left ventricular end diastolic pressure, a biphasic decrease then increase in coronary blood flow and bradycardia. Low-osmolar contrast media have less effect on these parameters, although Hexabrix produces more depression of left ventricular contraction during coronary arteriography than the other low-osmolar contrast media, probably because it contains sodium and meglumine. Low-osmolar contrast media also produce fewer electrocardiographic changes, including ventricular fibrillation.

Venous Thromboses Red Cell Effects:

When red cells are placed in a hypertonic medium, water leaves the interior of the cells by osmosis and they become more rigid.

Red blood cell rigidity or deformity is, thus, dependent on osmolarity and isosmolar solutions have no effect on red cell deformity.

Red cells that deform less easily are less able to pass through capillaries and may occlude them. When pulmonary arteries are already damaged, as in the Eisenmenger syndrome, injection of a hypertonic contrast medium into the pulmonary circulation may result in fatal pulmonary hypertension.

Increasing concentrations of contrast media have an increasing sickling effect on red cells in sickle cell anaemia.

Vascular Endothelial Damage:

Endothelial cells are liable to damage both by direct chemotoxicity and by the hyperosmolarity of contrast media. Contrast medium-induced thrombophlebitis is a particular complication of lower limb venography, but its incidence is reduced four-fold when low-osmolar contrast media are used in place of conventional high-osmolar contrast media.

Histamine Release:

Contrast media are capable of stimulating histamine release from mast cells and basophils and histamine has been implicated in the aetiology of adverse reactions. While hyperosmolarity is a factor, isomolar concentrations of contrast media will also stimulate histamine release and so the effect should be deemed chemotoxic.

Complement Effects:

Contrast media activate the complement series and a decrease in C_1-esterase inhibitor is also thought to be a factor in contrast media reactions. Low-osmolar contrast media have a lesser effect on complement activation.

Protein Binding and Enzyme Inhibition:

Contrast media are weakly protein bound and the degree of protein binding correlates with inhibition of the enzyme acetylcholinesterase.

Contrast medium side-effects such as vasodilatation, bradycardia, hypotension, bronchospasm and urticaria are all recognized cholinergic effects and may be related more to cholinesterase inhibition than osmolarity. The chemoreceptor trigger zone is situated in the lateral walls of the fourth ventricle and is unprotected by the blood-brain barrier. There is a cholinergic link between the chemoreceptor trigger zone and the emesis centre and the greater capacity of some contrast media to stimulate vomiting is probably a result of their greater ability to inhibit acetylcholinesterase.

Central Nervous System Effects:

Intravascular contrast media have an adverse effect on the central nervous system, particularly in those with an altered blood-brain barrier. Patients with cerebral tumours show an increased incidence of convulsions following enhancement for CT scans. Low-osmolar contrast media show less neurotoxicity. Ionic contrast media in the subarachnoid space cause seizures and arachnoiditis.

Pulmonary Effects:

Bronchospasm: Aetiology is uncertain but possible mechanisms include:

1. Direct histamine release from mast cells and platelets.
2. Cholinesterase inhibition.
3. Vagal overtone.
4. Complement activation.
5. Direct effect of contrast media on bronchi.

Bronchospasm is much less pronounced with iopamidol than with iothalamate.

Renal Effects:

Renal injury following injection of a conventional ionic contrast medium may be seen in 0.6% of hospitalized patients without pre-existing renal disease after urography and in 2% after arteriography. There are a number of predisposing factors:

1. Pre-existing impaired renal function.
2. Diabetes mellitus.
3. Dehydration.
4. Age—because of the greater incidence of cardiovascular disease in elderly.
5. Very large doses of contrast medium.

The mechanism of contrast medium-induced nephrotoxicity:

1. **Impaired renal perfusion:**
   a. Adverse cardiotoxic effects.
   b. Increased peripheral vasodilatation.
   c. Renal vascular bed changes (increased blood flow followed by a more prolonged decrease).
   d. Increased rigidity of red blood cells.
   e. Pre-dehydration.
   f. Osmotic diuresis.
2. **Glomerular injury:**
   a. Impaired perfusion.
   b. Hyperosmolar effects.
   c. Chemotoxic effects.
3. **Tubular injury:**
   a. Impaired perfusion.
   b. Hyperosmolar effects.
   c. Chemotoxic effects.
4. **Obstructive nephropathy:**
   a. Cytoplasmic vacuolation in tubules.
   b. Precipitation of Tamm-Horsfall protein.
   c. Precipitation of Bence Jones protein in multiple myeloma.

Indications for the Use of Low-Osmolar Contrast Media

The advantages of low-osmolar contrast media are:

1. More comfortable intravenous injections and arteriograms.
2. Less tissue toxicity.
3. Reduction in serious and fatal adverse reactions.

The following should receive low-osmolar contrast media:

1. Those at high risk from the hyperosmolar effects:
   a. Infants and small children.
   b. Those with renal and/or cardiac failure.
   c. Poorly hydrated patients.
   d. Patients with diabetes, myelomatosis or sickle cell anaemia.
   e. Patients who have had a previous severe anaphylactoid or allergic reaction to a conventional contrast medium or those with a strong allergic history.
2. Those who would suffer unnecessarily from the hyperosmolar effects of:
   a. Arteriograms under local anaesthetic.
   b. Various brand of contrast media in the market.

Urografin® 60%

Each ml contains:

Diatrizoic Acid anhydrous USP	471.78 mg
Meglumine USP	125.46 mg

Urografin® 76%

Each ml contains:

Diatrizoic Acid anhydrous USP	597.30 mg
Meglumine USP	159.24 mg

Trazogastro

Diatrizoic Acid salts

Meglumine salt	66% w/v
Sodium salt	10% w/v
In a flavoured aqueous base	
Iodine content	370 mg/ml

Normally the alimentary tract absorbs only minimal amounts of Trazogastro and no systemic effects follow its use.

When Trazogastro alone is used without the addition of barium sulphate, the hypertonicity of the high-concentrated solution may occasionally give rise to diarrhoea, but this ceases as soon as the intestine is emptied completely.

Indications of Trazogastro

Trazogastro is primarily indicated in cases in which the use of barium sulphate is unsatisfactory, undesirable, or contraindicated. Among these are:

- Suspected partial or complete stenosis.
- Acute haemorrhage.
- Threatening perforation (peptic, ulcer, diverticulum).
- Other acute conditions which are likely to require surgery.
- After resection of the stomach or intestine (danger of perforation or leak) Megacolon.
- Visualization of a foreign body or tumor before endoscopy.
- Visualization of a gastrocolic fistula.
- Apart from these conditions Trazogastro can generally be used for the same purposes as barium sulphate.

Oral Administration

In adult patients and children of 10 years of age and over, 60 ml are required for stomach and for a follow-through examination of 100 ml may be required. For elderly and cachectic patients a dilution with water in the proportion of 1:1 is recommended.

In children upto 10 years of age, 15 to 30 ml are generally sufficient. This dose can be diluted with water in the proportion of 1:1. For infants and debilitated small children it is recommended that the contrast medium be diluted with water in the proportion of 1:2.

Rectal Administration

For adult patients the contrast medium should be diluted with 3 to 4 times its volume of water not more than 500 ml of this diluted Trazogastro solution is required. For children over 5 years of age the contrast medium should be diluted with 4 to 5 times its volume of water, for children upto 5 years of age a dilution with water in the proportion of 1:5 is recommended.

Combination of Trazogastro with Barium Sulphate

In adult patients a ratio of approx. 30 ml. Trazogastro to the usual dose of barium has proved most satisfactory.

In children upto 10 years of age, 10 ml. Trazogastro may be added to the barium; in children upto 5 years of age, a ratio of 2 to 5 ml. Trazogastro to 100 ml barium has proved of value.

When Trazogastro alone is used, the dye generally reaches the rectum after 2 hours, Trazogastro barium-sulphate mixture may take upto 3 hours.

Computerised Tomography of the Abdomen

Trazogastro is used for the prevention of artifacts caused by air in the gastrointestinal tract. Demarcation of adjacent organs such as the pancreas in the scan picture has also been obtained.

500-1500 ml of diluted Trazogastro solution (about 3%) given orally.

Advantage

The use of Trazogastro does not endanger the patient even in case of intestinal obstruction or pyloric stenosis, or in cases of perforation or leakage. No damage is done if Trazogastro enters the peritoneal cavity.

Since the aqueous solution of Trazogastro leaves no deposit or opaque residue, endoscopy can be performed immediately after the radiological investigation.

In cases of acute haemorrhage Trazogastro while outlining the mucosal pattern, flows around the blood clot and makes it possible to locate the site of the haemorrhage.

NON-IONIC CONTRAST MEDIUM

Iopamidol Injection

1. **Lek-Pamidol 300**

   Each ml contains:

   Iopamidol USP 612.4 mg

   Equivalent to 300 mg of Iodine

   Water for Injection IP q.s.

   Tromethamine USP 1 mg per ml as buffer and Edetate Calcium Disodium USP (on anhydrous basis) 0.3 mg per ml as stabilizer.

2. **Lek-Pamidol 370**

   Each ml contains:

   Iopamidol USP 755.3 mg

   Equivalent to 370 mg of Iodine

   Water for Injection IP q.s.

   Tromethamine USP 1 mg per ml as buffer and Edetate Calcium Disodium USP (on anhydrous basis) 0.37 mg per ml as stabilizer.

Iopamidol is an Angiography contrast medium of the new generation of non-ionic compounds, which are water-soluble because its molecular structure incorporates hydrophilic groups.

General Indications

Angiography: Cerebral arteriography, coronary arteriography, thoracic aortography, abdominal aortography, angiocardiography, selective visceral arteriography, peripheral arteriography, venography, digital subtraction angiography (DSA), DSA of cerebral arteries, DSA of peripheral arteries, DSA of abdominal arteries.

Contraindications

There are no definite or absolute contraindications to the use of iopamidol, with the possible exception of Waldenstrom's macroglobulinemia, multiple myeloma, and severe liver and kidney diseases.

Do not mix any other drugs with contrast medium solutions.

Dose

Angiography

	Concentration (mg iodine/ml)
Cerebral arteriography	300
Coronary arteriography	370
Thoracic aortography	370
Abdominal aortography	370
Angiocardiography	370
Selective visceral arteriography	300-370
Peripheral arteriography	300-370
Digital subtraction angiography	300-370
Venography	300

CONTRAST MEDIUM FOR MRI

Omniscan™

(Gadodiamide)

Each 1 ml injection contains as active ingredient 287 mg gadodiamide (GdDTPA-BMA) equivalent to 0.5 mmol/ml. Other ingredients are: caldiamide sodium, sodium hydroxide 1 M or hydrochloric acid 1 M and water for injections.

Non-ionic paramagnetic contrast medium for cranial and spinal magnetic resonance imaging (MRI) in adults for intravenous administration.

The product provides contrast enhancement and facilitates visualization of abnormal structures or lesions in the CNS.

Gadodiamide does not cross the intact blood brain barrier. Administration of Omniscan causes signal enhancement from areas where blood brain barrier dysfunction has been induced by pathological processes, and may provide greater diagnostic yield than unenhanced MRI. Lack of enhancement need not indicate absence of pathology since some types of low grade malignancies or inactive MS-plaques fail to enhance; it can be used for differential diagnosis between different pathologies.

Gadodiamide is rapidly distributed in the extracellular fluid. The volume of distribution is equivalent to that of extracellular water. The distribution half life is approximately 4 minutes and the elimination half-time is approximately 70 minutes.

Gadodiamide is excreted through the kidneys by glomerular filtration. Approximately 85% of the administered dose is recovered in the urine by 4 hours and 95-98% by 24 hours after intravenous injection.

The recommended dosage is 0.1 mmol/kg body weight (equivalent to 0.2 ml/kg b.w.) upto 100 kg. Above 100 kg body weight 20 ml is usually sufficient to provide diagnostically adequate contrast.

Contraindications

Omniscan should not be used in patients known to have hypersensitivity to Omniscan or its constituents.

Precaution

Anaphylactic shock, hypersensitivity reactions (urticaria and other possible allergic phenomenon) may occur.

Side Effect

Discomfort with general sensation of warmth, coolness or a sensation of local pressure or pain at the injection site are occasionally seen. Others are dizziness, nausea, headache and a perverted sensation of taste or smell, urticaria, itching or an irritation in the throat, vomiting or somnolence, transient renal failure.

Other Informations

Osmolality (mOsm/kg H_2O) at 37°C	780
Viscosity (mPa.s) at 20°C	2.8
Viscosity (mPa.s) at 37°C	1.9
Density at 20°C (kg/1)	1.15
Molar Relaxivity	
r_1 ($mM^{-1}.s^{-1}$) at 10 MHz and 37°C	4.6
r_2 ($mM^{-1}.s^{-1}$) at 10 MHz and 37°C	5.1

pH 6.0-7.0.

GASTROINTESTINAL TRACT

Methods for Demonstration of GIT

1. Plain film.
2. Barium swallow.

3. Barium meal.
4. Barium follow-through.
5. Small bowel enema.
6. Barium enema.
7. Radioisotope-99 mTc study for Meckel's diverticulum.
8. Arteriography.
9. CT.

Barium Swallow

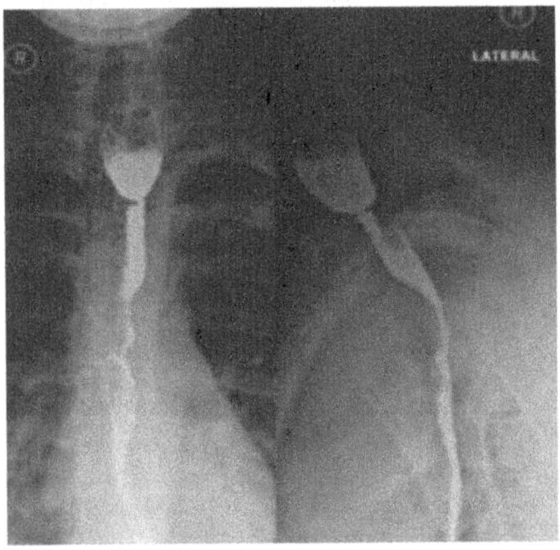

Fig. 3.2: Barium swallow esophagus (Esophogram)

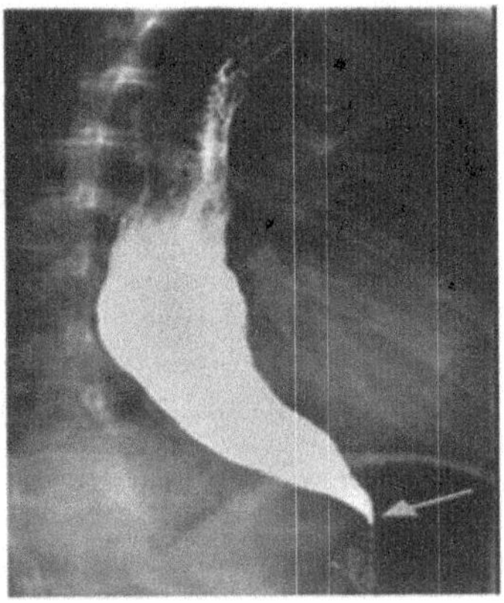

Fig. 3.3: Barium swallow esophagus in a case cardia achalasia (arrow)

Indications:

1. Dysphagia.
2. Pain in chest.
3. Tracheoesophageal fistula in children.
4. Left atrial enlargement.
5. Preoperative assessment of carcinoma of bronchus.
6. Assessment of site of perforation:

   Contraindication .... None

   Patient preparation .... None

   Preliminary film .... None

Technique:

1. Patient is in erect RAO position to throw the esophagus clear of spine. An ample mouthful of barium is swallowed and spot films of the upper and lower esophagus are taken. Oesophageal varices are better seen in prone RPO position, as they will be more distended.
2. If rapid serial radiography is required, it may be performed in right lateral, RAO and PA position.
3. To demonstrate a tracheoesophageal fistula in infants a fine nasogastric tube is introduced to the level of mid-esophagus, and the diluted barium is injected through syringe into distended esophagus. This will allow the barium to pass through any small fistula that may be present. It is important to take radiographs, in the lateral position, simultaneously with the injection of barium, for otherwise the fistula may be missed.

   The barium is introduced through a nasogastric tube because infants might reflux it into the trachea if swallowing from a bottle. It would not then be possible to determine whether its presence in the bronchi was due to a small fistula that was difficult to see or due to aspirate. The use of a nasogastric tube bypasses the swallowing mechanism.

Barium Meal

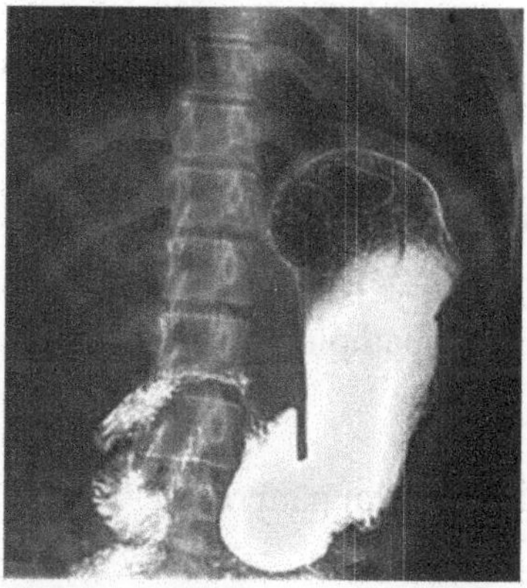

Fig. 3.4: Barium meal for stomach and duodenum

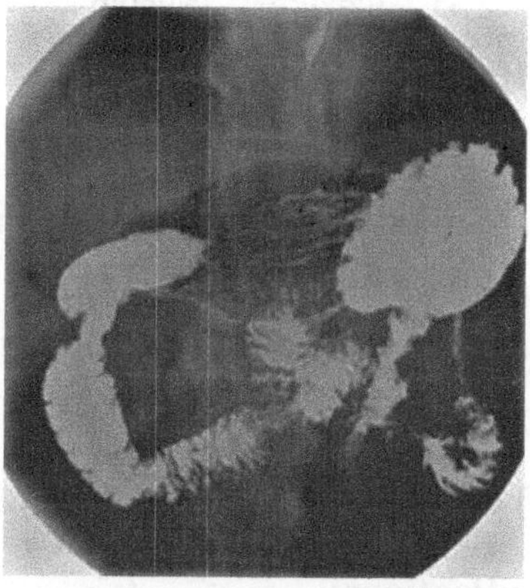

Fig. 3.5: Barium meal showing duodenal loop

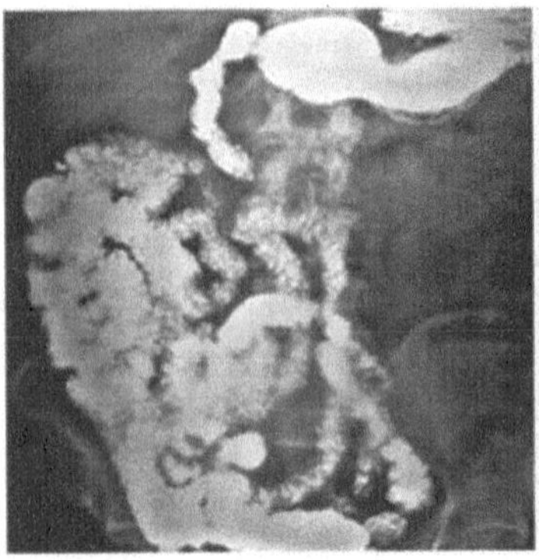

Fig. 3.6: Barium meal study showing small intestine

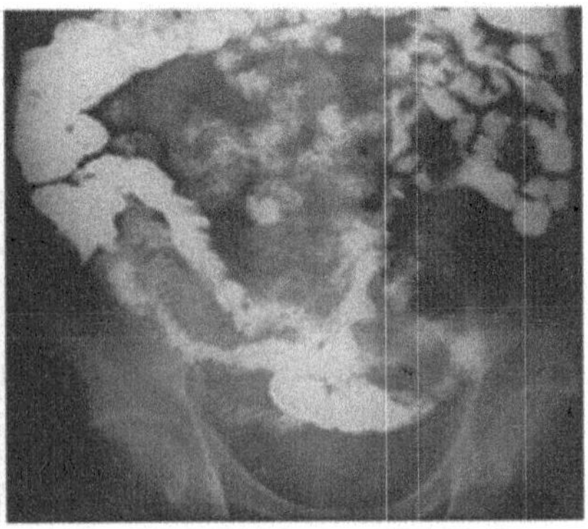

Fig. 3.7: Barium meal showing ileocaecal area

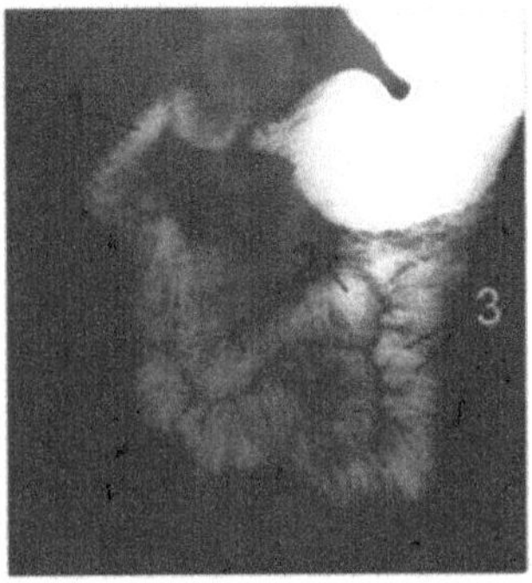

Fig. 3.8: Barium meal upper GIT
1. C-loop Duodenum
2. D.J. Flexure 3. Jejunum

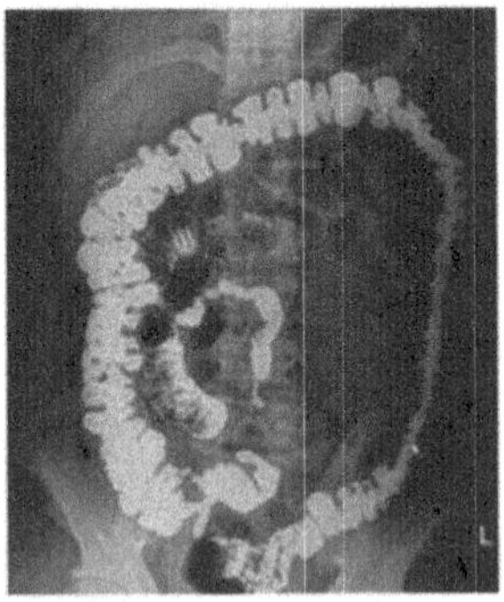

Fig. 3.9: Barium meal follow-through study

Methods:

Single Contrast

1. Children—Since it usually is not necessary to demonstrate mucosal pattern.
2. Very ill adults—To demonstrate gross pathology only.

Double Contrast

The method of choice to demonstrate mucosal pattern.

Indications:

1. Dyspepsia.

2. Weight loss.
3. Upper abdominal mass.
4. GI haemorrhage.
5. Unexplained iron deficiency anaemia.
6. Partial obstruction.
7. Assessment of site of perforation.

Contraindication:

Complete large bowel obstruction.

Patient Preparation:

1. Nil orally for 6 hours prior to examination.
2. Patient must not smoke on the day of the examination as this causes increased gastric mobility.
3. It should be ensured that there are no contraindications to the pharmacological agents used.

Preliminary Film—None.

Technique:

Double Contrast Method

1. A gas producing agent is swallowed. The requirements of these agents are as follows:
   i. Production of an adequate volume of gas 200-400 ml.
   ii. Non-interference with barium coating.
   iii. No-bubble production.
   iv. Rapid dissolution, leaving no residue.
   v. Easily swallowed.
   vi. Low cost.
2. The patient then drinks the barium while lying on his left side, supported by his elbow. This position prevents the barium from reaching the duodenum quickly and so obscuring the greater curvature of stomach.

3. The patient then lies supine and slightly on his right side, to bring the barium up against the gastroesophageal junction. This manoeuvre is screened to check the reflux, which may be revealed by asking the patient to cough or to swallow water while in this position. The significance of reflux produced by tipping the patient's head down is debatable, as this is an unphysiological position. If reflux is observed, spot films are taken to record the level to which it ascends.
4. I.V. Buscopan (smooth muscle relaxant) 20 mg in 1 amp is given.
5. The patient is asked to roll onto his right side and then quickly over in a complete circle, to finish in an RAO position. This role is performed to coat the gastric mucosa with barium.

Films:

1. Spot films of stomach (lying)
   a. RAO—to demonstrate the antrum and greater curve.
   b. Supine—to demonstrate the antrum and body.
   c. LAO—to demonstrate lesser curve on face.
   d. Left lateral tilted, head up 45° to demonstrate the fundus.

   From the left lateral position the patient returns to a supine position and then rolls onto his left side and over into a prone position. This sequence of movement is required to avoid barium flooding into the duodenal loop, which would occur if the patient were to roll onto his right side to achieve a prone position.
2. Spot film of the duodenum loop (lying)
   a. Prone—the patient lies on a compression pad to prevent barium from flooding into the duodenum.
   b. To demonstrate anterior wall of duodenal loop RAO film may be taken.
3. Spot films of duodenal cap (lying)
   a. Prone
   b. RAO

c. Supine

d. LAO.

4. Additional views of the fundus in an erect position may be taken at this stage, if there is suspicion of a fundal lesion.
5. Spot film of oesophagus are taken, while barium is being swallowed, to complete the examination.

After Care

1. The patient should be warned that his bowel motion will be white for a few days after the examination, and to keep his bowels open, laxatives may be added to avoid barium impaction, which can be painful.
2. The patient must not leave the department until any blurring of vision produced by Buscopan has resolved.

Complications

1. Leakage of barium from an unsuspected perforation.
2. Aspiration.
3. Conversion of a partial large bowel obstruction into a complete obstruction by the impaction of barium.
4. Barium appendicitis, if barium impacts in the appendix.
5. Side-effects of the pharmacological agents used.

Barium Meal Follow-through

Methods:

1. Single contrast.
2. In the investigation of suspected disaccharidase deficiency, the examination is performed first without, and then with 25 gm of appropriate sugar added to the barium.

3. Enhanced with an effervescent agent.
4. Enhanced with a pneumocolon technique.

Indications:

1. Pain.
2. Diarrhoea.
3. Bleeding.
4. Partial obstruction.

Contraindications:

1. Complete obstruction.
2. Suspected perforation.

Patient Preparation:

1. A laxative on the evening prior to the examination.
2. Metoclopramide 20 mg orally 20 min before the examination.

Preliminary Film

Plain abdominal film.

Technique:

The aim is to deliver a single column of barium into the small bowel. This is achieved by lying the patient on his right side after the barium has been ingested. The metoclopramide enhances the rate of gastric emptying. If the transit time through the small bowel is still found to be slow, a dry meal may help to speed up.

Films:

1. Prone PA films of the abdomen are taken every 20 minutes during 1st hour, and subsequently every 30 minutes until the colon is reached. The prone position is mixed because the pressure on the abdomen help to separate the loops of small intestine.

2. Spot films of the terminal ileum are taken in supine position. A compression pad is used to displace any overlapping loops of small bowel that are obscuring the terminal ileum.

Additional Films:

1. To separate loops of small intestine:
   a. Oblique.
   b. With X-ray tube angled to the pelvis.
   c. With the patient tilted head down.
2. To determine diverticulum:

   Erect—This position will reveal any fluid level caused by contrast medium retained within the diverticula.

After Care

As for barium meal.

Complications

As for barium meal.

Small Bowel Enema

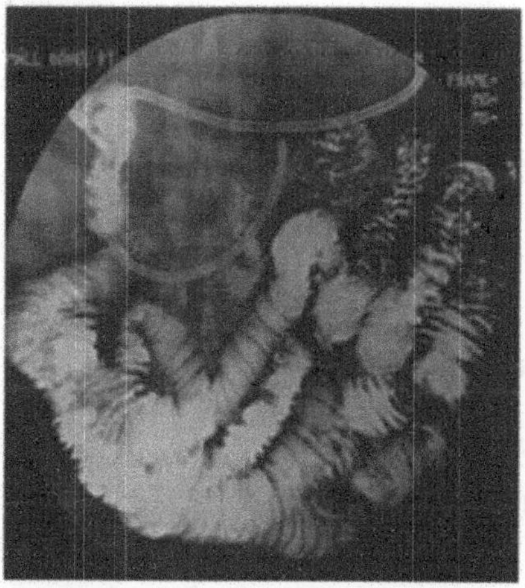

Fig. 3.10: Small bowel enema through Bilbao – Dotter tube

Advantage:

This procedure gives better visualisation of the small bowel than that achieved by a barium followthrough because rapid infusion of a large continuous column of contrast medium directly into the jejunum avoids segmentation of the barium column and does not allow time for flocculation to occur.

Disadvantage:

Intubation may be unpleasant for the patient, and may prove difficult. It is also time-consuming for the radiologists.

Indications and Contraindications:

Same as for barium follow through.

Contrast Medium

Micropaque 100% w/v.

This is diluted with tap water to give a volume of 1000 ml with a Sp Gr of 1.3. This reduced viscosity produces better mucosal coating and the reduced density permits the visualisation of bowel loops which may otherwise have been obscured by a denser contrast medium in an overlying loop.

An alternative way to gain a double contrast effect is to use a small (100 ml) bolus of micropaque followed by a continuous infusion of methyl cellulose (100 ml of cologel made up of 2 liters with distilled water).

Equipment:

Bilbao-Dotter tube with guidewire.

Patient's Preparation:

1. Low residue diet and laxatives for 2 days prior to the examination.
2. If the patient is taking any antispasmodic drugs, they must be stopped 1 day prior to the examination.

3. Amethocain Lozenge 30 mg, 30 mt before the examination.
4. Immediately before the examination the Pharynx is anaesthesized with Lignocaine spray.

Preliminary Film:

Plain abdominal film.

Techniques:

1. The patient sits on the edge of the X-ray table. After the pharynx is anaesthetised, the tube is passed through the nose/mouth and advanced into the stomach.
2. The patient then lies on his left side so that the gastric air bubble rises into the antrum, so straightening out the stomach. This allows the tube to be passed more easily into the duodenum. However, if the tube is not passing through the pylorus, the guidewire is introduced in order to give it some rigidity and then it is advanced with a clockwise rotational movement. Firm pressure on the greater curvature of the stomach by a lead gloved hand also facilitates passage into the duodenum by preventing the formation of a large loop into the stomach when the tube is advanced. Rotating the patient to the erect position will help overcome any tendency of the tube to coil in the fundus of stomach. If difficulty is still encountered, metoclopramide (20 mp I.V.) still may be injected to encourage its passage.
3. When the tip of the tube has been passed through the pylorus, the guidewire is withdrawn and the tube is advanced to the level of the ligament of Treitz, at the distal end of 4th part of duodenum. This is to diminish the risk of aspiration due to reflux of barium into the stomach in conjunction with an anaesthetized pharynx.
4. Barium is then run in quickly, and spot films are taken of barium column and its leading edge at the region of interest, until the colon is reached. If methyl cellulose is used, it is infused continuously, after an initial bolus of 100 ml of barium, until the barium has reached the colon.

5. Then the tube is withdrawn, aspirating any residual fluid in the stomach. This is to decrease the risk of aspiration.
6. Finally, prone and supine abdominal films were taken.

After Care

1. Nil orally for 5 hours after the procedure.
2. Patient should be warned that diarrhoea may occur as a result of the large volume of fluid given.

Complication

1. Aspiration.
2. Perforation of the bowel owing to manipulation of the guidewire.

Barium Enema

Methods:

Single Contrast:

a. *Children*—Since it is usually not necessary to demonstrate mucosal pattern.
b. Reduction of an intussusception.

Double Contrast:

The method of choice to demonstrate mucosal pattern.

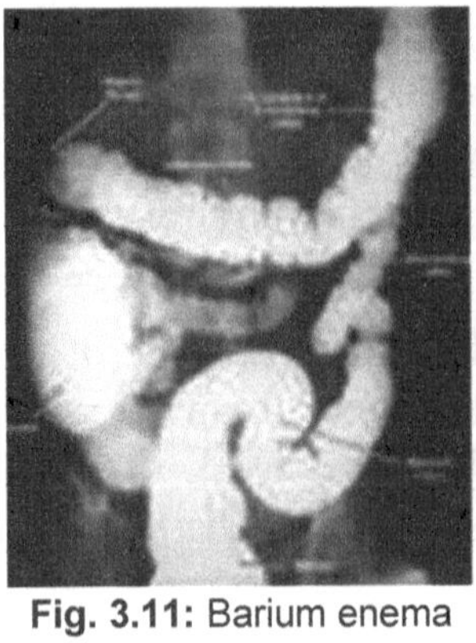

Fig. 3.11: Barium enema (Single contrast)

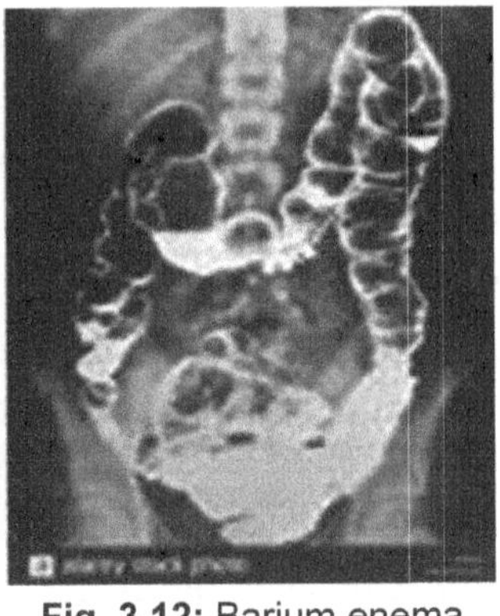

Fig. 3.12: Barium enema (Double contrast)

Indications:

1. Change in bowel habit.
2. Pain.
3. Mass.
4. Melena.
5. Obstruction.

Contraindications:

Absolute:

1. Toxic megacolon.
2. Pseudomembranous colitis.
3. Rectal biopsy within the previous 3 days (it is preferable to wait for 7 days).

Relative:

1. Incomplete bowel preparation.
2. Recent Barium meal.

Equipments:

Miller disposable enema tube is needed. If the patient is incontinent, it is permissible to use a tube with an inflatable cuff. However, its use should be confined to such cases, owing to the increased risk of perforation.

Patient Preparation:

Many regimens for bowel preparation have been reviewed (Dodds *et al.,* 1977, Kendrick *et al.,* 1981, Bartram *et al.,* 1984).

For 3 days prior to examination: Low residue diet.

On the day prior to examination:

1. Fluids only.
2. Picolax—At 8.00 AM to 6.00 PM.

On the day of the examination:

A high colonic washout with 2 litres of tap water is given. The patient then empties his bowels. At least 1 hour must elapse before starting the barium enema to allow for the colon to absorb the excess water. <0.25% of Tannic acid may be used in saline enema to promote evacuation. It should not be used in case of hepatic failure or inflammatory bowel diseases.

Preliminary Film:

Plain Abdominal Film:

a. To assess bowel preparation.
b. To exclude toxic megacolon.

Technique:

Double Contrast:

1. The patient lies on his side on a rubber sheet. The catheter is inserted gently into the rectum. Connections are made to the barium reservoir and the hand pump for injecting air.
2. I.V. Buscopan 20 mg.
3. Infusion of barium is commenced. Intermittent screening is required to check the progress of the barium. The infusion is terminated when the barium has reached the splenic flexure.
4. Air is then gently pumped round towards the caecum, and producing the double contrast effect.
5. From the prone position, the patient rolls onto his left side and over into RAO position so that the barium coats the bowel mucosa.

Films:

1. Spot films of rectum and sigmoid colon (lying):
   - RAO
   - Prone

- LPO
- Left lateral of rectum.

2. Spot films of hepatic flexure, splenic flexure and rectum (erect):
   - LAO to open out the splenic flexure.
   - RAO to open out the hepatic flexure.
   - Right lateral of rectum.
3. Spot film of caecum (lying). Positioning of the patient supine, lying slightly on the right side and with a slight head down tilt which usually give a double contrast effect in the caecum. Some compression with a lead-gloved hand may be necessary to persuade a stubborn pool of barium out of caecal pole.
4. Over couch films are required to demonstrate the large bowel (lying)
   - Supine
   - Prone
   - Left lateral decubitus
   - Right lateral decubitus
   - Prone with tube angled 45° caudal and centred 5 cm above the posterior superior iliac spines. This separates overlying loops of sigmoid colon.

After Care

1. The patient should be warned that his bowel motions will be white for a few days after the examination, and to keep his bowels open with laxatives to avoid barium impaction, which may be painful.
2. The patient must not leave the department until any blurring of vision produced by Buscopan has reached.

Complications

1. Perforation of the bowel. There is an increased risk of this in:
   a. Infants and the elderly.

b. Obstructing neoplasm.
c. Ulceration of bowel wall.
d. Inflation of a Foley catheter balloon in a colostomy or rectum.
e. Patient on steroid therapy.
f. Hypothyroidism.

2. Venous extravasation: Pulmonary embolism—Death in 80%.
3. Water intoxication (Drowsiness and convulsions). Increased risk of megacolon because of large area of bowel mucosa available for absorption of water.
4. Intramural barium.
5. Cardiac arrhythmia due to rectal distension.
6. Transient bacteriemia.
7. Side effects of pharmacological agents used.

Instant Barium Enema

This is preferred in inflammatory bowel disease of colon. This is done without bowel preparation as the bowel does not contain fecal residue.

Indication:

To show the extent and severity of mucosal lesions in active ulcerative colitis.

Contraindication:

1. Toxic megacolon.
2. Rectal biopsy within previous 3 days.
3. Long standing ulcerative colitis.
4. Crohn's colitis.

Preliminary Film:

Plain abdominal film to exclude toxic megacolon.

Technique:

As for normal barium enema.

Films:

1. Prone.
2. Left lateral decubitus.
3. Erect.

Barium Enema Reduction of an Intussusception:

This procedure should be done under surgical consultation.

Contraindications:

1. Evidence of peritonitis or perforation.
2. Advanced intestinal obstruction.

Patient's Preparation:

1. Sedation with papaveretum 0.2 mg/kg.
2. Correction of fluid and electrolyte imbalance.

Preliminary Film:

Plain abdominal film to assess bowel distension and to exclude perforation.

Technique:

1. 16-22 F Foley catheter is inserted into the rectum and buttocks taped rightly together to provide a seal. It is usually necessary to inflate the balloon and this should be performed under fluoroscopic control so that the rectum is not distended.
2. The child is positioned supine and disturbed as little as possible during the procedure.
3. The bag containing barium is raised to 100 cm above the table top to provide gentle hydrostatic pressure and barium is run in. Progress of the column of barium is monitored by intermittent fluoroscopy.

4. Intussusception is reduced and is only considered complete when the terminal ileum fills with barium.
5. If the intussusception does not move after 5 minutes of sustained pressure, the barium is run out and the child rested for 5 minutes. A second attempt is then made of reduction, ceases again, a third attempt is made, but if this does not succeed, the intussusception is considered irreducible and arrangements are made for surgery.

Films:

1. Spot films as required.
2. Post-reduction film.

Complication

Perforation.

After Care

Observation in hospital for 24 hours.

Therapeutic Gastrografin Enema in Meconium Ileus

Prior to this procedure a diagnostic barium enema is performed to exclude other forms of intestinal obstruction.

Contraindications:

1. Perforation.
2. Volvulus.

Patient's Preparation:

1. The baby must be well hydrated prior to the procedure as there may be considerable fluid loss into the bowel, and an I.V. saline drip is mandatory.
2. Antibiotic cover.

Technique:

The aim is to run a hypertonic water-soluble contrast medium through the colon and into the small bowel to surround the meconium. The hypertonic contrast medium draws water into the bowel and so helps to dislodge the sticky meconium. If successful, meconium should be passed in the next hour. If no result is seen even after 1 hour, the procedure is deemed to have failed and surgical intervention will be necessary because prolonged contact of a hyperosmolar solution with the bowel mucosa can cause necrosis. If the passage of meconium is incomplete, a second enema may be required.

Sinogram

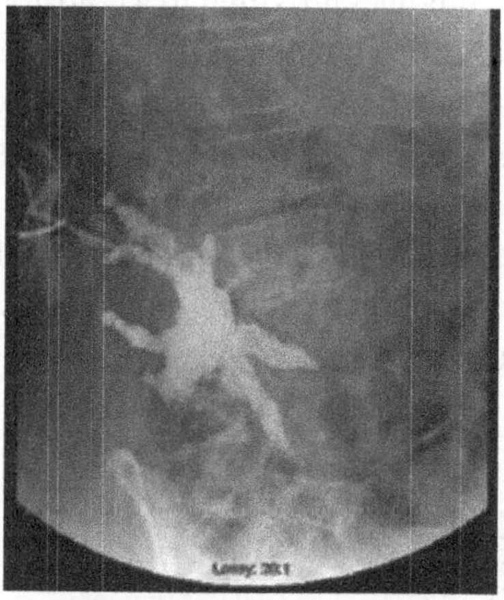

Fig. 3.13: Sinogram

A water soluble contrast medium is used unless there is any suspicion of a connection with the cavity, in such a case Dinosil aqueous is safe alternative. A preliminary film is taken to exclude the presence of opaque foreign body. A fine catheter is than inserted into the orifice of the sinus, next to which a metal marker has been placed. After a gauze pad has been firmly placed over the orifice to discourage reflux, the contrast medium is injected under fluoroscopic control. Spot films are taken in AP and Lat. and Oblique position.

Loopogram

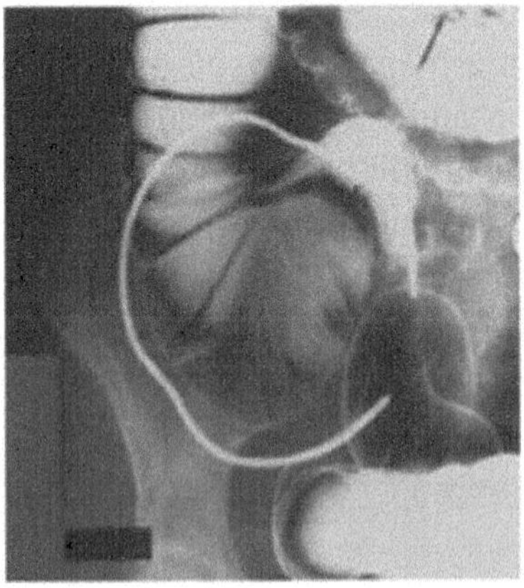

Fig. 3.14: Loopogram

This investigation of bowel proximal to a colostomy is performed by inserting the tip of a Foley's catheter for a few cm only into appropriate stoma. The balloon may be inflated carefully within the lumen of bowel proximal to stoma to provide a seal. The barium is run into bowel and spot films are taken. The bowel distal to colostomy may be investigated by barium run in the rectum in the usual manner. Water-soluble medium should be used if breakdown in anastomosis is under suspicion.

Fistulogram

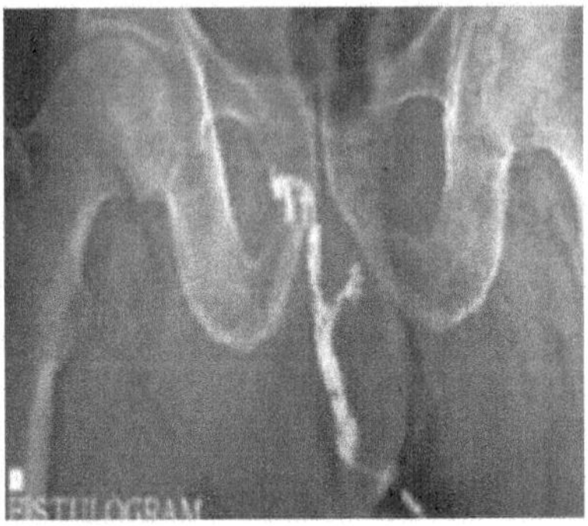

Fig. 3.15: Fistulogram

Fine plastic tube according to opening of fistulous tract is placed through opening. Water soluble contrast media is injected under fluoroscopic control, when the tract is visualised. Than AP, Lat, obl. Views are obtained. This will show both end of the tract.

Biliary Tract and Pancreas

Methods to Demonstrate Gallbladder and Biliary Tract:

1. Plain abdomen skiagram.
2. Oral cholecystography.
3. Intravenous choledochography or cholangiography.
4. Operative cholangiography.
5. T-tube cholangiography.
6. Endoscopic retrograde cholangiopancreaticography (ERCP).
7. Percutaneous transhepatic cholangiography (PTC).
8. Ultrasound.
9. Radioisotope study:
   - 99mTc-HiDA, BiDA or PIPIDA.
   - I^{123}-BSP ^{131}I-Rose-Bengal.
10. C.T.
11. M.R.C.P. (Magnetic resonance cholangiopancreaticography).

Methods to Demonstrate Pancreas:

1. Plain abdomen skiagram.
2. Hypotonic duodenography.
3. Endoscopic retrograde pancreaticography (ERP).
4. Arteriography
   - Coeliac axis.
   - Superior mesenteric artery.
5. Venography
   - Percutaneous transhepatic method.
   - Umbilical vein catheterization.

6. Radioisotope study—^{75}selenomethionine—demonstrate normal pancreas.
7. USG.
8. CT.
9. MRI.

With advances in ultrasonography and MRI equipments, oral cholecystography, I.V. cholangiogram, operative cholangiogram are stopped completely. For pancreatic pathology, USG, CT and MRI are preferred investigations.

T-Tube Cholangiography

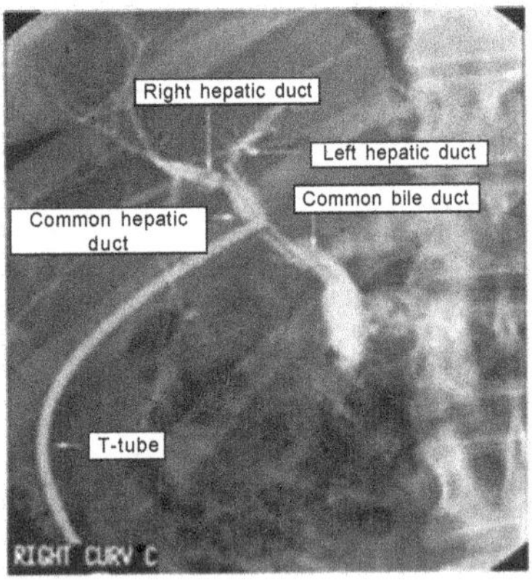

Fig. 3.16: T- tube cholangiogram

Indications—To exclude biliary tract calculi where:

1. Operative cholangiogram was not performed.
2. Results of operative cholangiogram are not satisfactory or are suspect (left over calculus).

Contraindications—None.

Contrast Media—Water soluble contrast media.

Equipment—Fluoroscopy X-ray unit with spot film device.

Patient Preparation—Nil.

Preliminary Film—Supine AP abdomen for right quadrant.

Technique:

1. Examination is performed on or about the 10th post operative day, prior to pulling out the T-tube.
2. Patient lies supine on X-ray table. The drainage tube is clamped off near the patient's skin and cleaned thoroughly with antiseptic.
3. A 20 G needle is inserted through tube proximal to clamp then contrast medium is injected under fluoroscopic control, the total volume of contrast medium depends upon filling of duct.

Films:

10" × 12" under spot film device:

PA, RAO, LAO.

After Care:

None.

Complications

Due to Contrast Medium—The biliary ducts do absorb contrast medium and cholangiovenous reflex can occur with injection at high pressure, adverse reactions are therefore possible but the incidence is small.

Due to Technique—Injection of contrast medium under high pressure into an obstructed biliary tract can produce septicaemia.

Percutaneous Transhepatic Cholangiogram

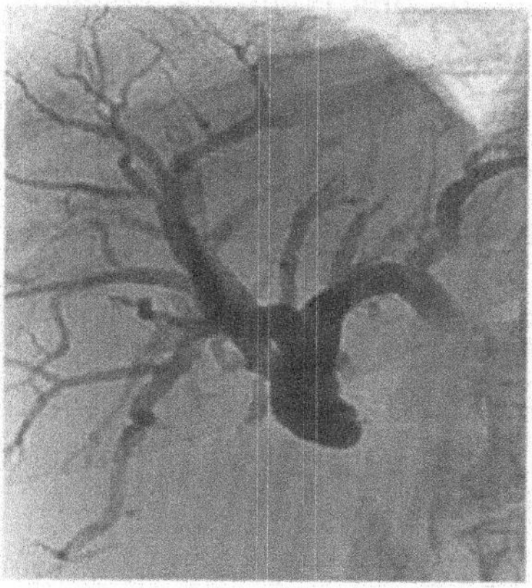

Fig. 3.17: Percutaneous transhepatic cholangiogram (P.T.C.)

Indication—Undiagnosed jaundice.

Contraindications:

1. Bleeding tendency.
2. Biliary tract sepsis.
3. Non-availability of prompt surgical facilities.
4. Hydatid cyst.

Contrast Medium—Water soluble contrast medium.

Equipment:

1. Fluoroscopic X-ray unit with spot film device.
2. Chiba needle (Fine, flexible 22G needle 18 cm long).

Patient Preparation:

1. Hb, prothrombin time and platelet count are to be evaluated and corrected if necessary.
2. Prophylactic antibiotic.
3. Nil orally for 5 hours before examination.
4. Premedication.

Preliminary Film:

Supine AP film right upper quadrant of abdomen.

Technique:

1. Patient lies supine, under fluoroscopic control, a metal marker is placed on the skin in the right sided mid-axillary line such that its position overlies the liver during full inspiration and expiration.
2. Using aseptic technique the skin, deeper tissues and liver capsule are anaesthesized at the site of metal marker.
3. During suspended respiration, the chiba needle is inserted into the liver. Once it is within the liver parenchyma, the patient is allowed shallow respiration. It is advanced parallel to the table top in the direction of xiphisternum until just short of right lateral margin of spine.

4. The stilet is withdrawn and needle connected to contrast filled syringe and under fluoroscopic guidance the contrast media is injected while the needle is slowly withdrawn. If duct is not entered, at the first attempt, the needle tip is withdrawn to approximately 2-3 cm from the liver capsule and further advanced or withdrawal are made, directing the needle tip more cranially, caudally, anteriorly or posteriorly until duct is entered. If a duct has not been entered after ten attempts, the procedure is terminated and the assumption is made that the ducts are not dilated.
5. Excessive parenchymal injection should be avoided and when it does occur, it results in opacification of intrahepatic lymphatics. Injection of contrast medium into a vein or artery is followed by rapid dispersion.
6. If the intrahepatic ducts are seen to be dilated, bile should be aspirated and sent for microbiological examination.
7. Contrast medium is injected to fill up the duct system and define the lower end of an obstruction. The needle is then withdrawn.
8. Puncture site is sealed with tinc benzoin or Healex.

Films:

PA, 45° RAO, Rt. and Lt. lateral, trendelenburg, spot film of GB. Delayed film.

After Care

Patient should be observed for 6 hours about pulse and BP.

Complications

Morbidity approx. 5%, mortality <1%.

Due to Contrast Medium:

Allergic or idiosyncratic reaction.

Due to Technique:

Local:

- Puncture of extrahepatic structure.
- Intrathoracic injection.
- Cholangitis.
- Bile leak.
- Subphrenic abscess.
- Haemorrhage.
- Shock.

Generalised:

- Bacteriemia.
- Septicaemia.
- Endotoxic shock.

ERCP

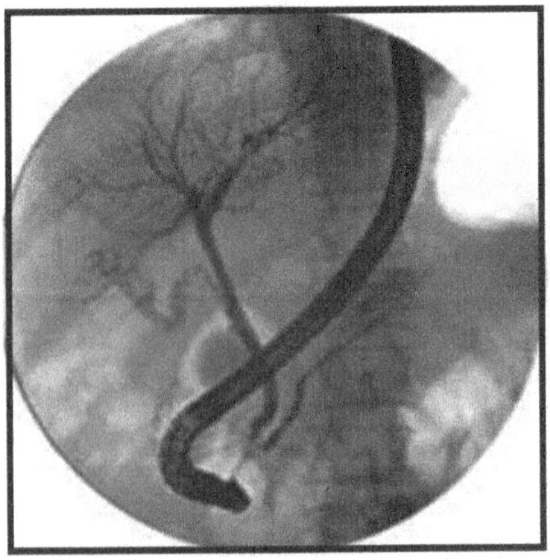

Fig. 3.18: Endoscopic retrocholangiopancreaticography (E.R.C.P.)

Indications:

1. Examination of extrahepatic biliary obstruction.

2. Post cholecystectomy syndrome.
3. Investigation of diffuse biliary disease.
4. Pancreatic disease.

Contraindications:

1. Australia antigen +ve.
2. AIDS +ve.
3. Oesophageal obstruction, varices, pyloric stenosis.
4. Previous gastric surgery.
5. Acute pancreatitis.
6. Pancreatic pseudocyst.
7. When glucagon/buscopan are contraindicated.
8. Severe cardiorespiratory diseases.

Contrast Medium:

Water soluble contrast medium.

Equipments:

- Side viewing endoscope.
- Polyethylene catheter.
- Fluoroscopic X-ray unit with spot film device.

Patient's Preparation:

1. Nil orally for 4 hours prior to procedure.
2. Premedication—Pethidine, Atropine.
3. Antibiotic cover.

Preliminary Film:

Prone AP/LAO of upper abdomen to cheque for opaque gallstones and pancreatic calcification/calculi.

Technique:

The pharynx is anesthetized with 2% xylocain spray then the patient is given diazepam 5 mg slow I.V. He, then, lies on his left side and endoscope is introduced. The ampulla of Vater is located and the patient is turned prone. A polyethylene catheter profiled with contrast medium is inserted into ampulla, having ensured that all air bubbles are excluded. As small test injection of contrast under fluoroscopic control is made to determine the position of canula. Avoid overfilling of pancreas. If biliary obstruction is present then bile should be sent for culture and sensitivity.

Film:

Prone, both posterior oblique views.

Bile Ducts:

1. Early filling films to show calculi.
   a. Prone—Straight and post oblique.
   b. Supine—Straight both oblique, trendelenburg to fill intrahepatic ducts, semi-erect to fill lower end of CBD and GB.
2. Films following removal of endoscope.
3. Delayed film to assess the GB and emptying of CBD.

After Care

1. Nil orally until sensation has returned to the pharynx (½–3 hours).
2. Pulse, Temp, BP ½ hourly × 6 hours.
3. Antibiotic.
4. Serum/urinary amylase if pancreatitis is suspected.

Complications

Due to Contrast Medium:

1. Allergic reaction.
2. Acute pancreatitis—with large volume and at high pressure injection.

Due to Technique:

Local—Damage by endoscope, rupture of esophagus, damage to ampulla, proxy pancreatic duct and distal common duct.

Distant—Bacteriemia, septicaemia, aspiration pneumonitis, hyperamylasaemia, acute pancreatitis.

Percutaneous Extraction of Retained Calculi (Burhenne Technique)

Indications:

Retained biliary calculi seen on T-tube cholangiogram.

Contraindications:

1. Small T-tube (< 12F).
2. Tortuous T-tube course in soft tissue.
3. Acute pancreatitis.
4. Drain in situ.

Contrast Medium:

Water soluble contrast medium.

Equipment:

Fluoroscopic X-ray unit with spot film device.

Med-tech steerable catheter system with wire baskets.

Patient's Preparation:

1. T-tube should be greater than 12F.
2. T-tube should be brought out obliquely towards the Rt. flank.
3. Following discovery of retained stone on the 10th P.O. day on T-tube cholangiogram, the patient should be discharged with

T-tube clamped for at least 4 weeks to allow the formation of a solid fistulous tract.

4. Hospitalisation one day prior to procedure.
5. Prophylactic antibiotic and premedication 1 hour prior to procedure.
6. Analgesia during procedure.

Technique:

1. Patient lies supine on X-ray table. T-tube cholangiogram is performed to accurately localize the retained calculus.
2. T-tube is slowly withdrawn from the patient.
3. A steerable catheter is advanced down the T-tube track and its tip is positioned just beyond the calculus. A basket is then inserted through the catheter and opened beyond the stone. The opened basket and catheter are then slowly withdrawn and stone engaged. The basket should not be closed as the stone may be dislodged or fragmented. The catheter system with the engaged stone in the basket should be slowly withdrawn to the skin surface in one movement.
4. The duct system is opacified by intermittent injection of contrast through the steerable catheter.
5. At the end of procedure a suction catheter is manipulated into the duct system and sutured to the skin.
6. Stone upto 10 mm in diam may be extracted through 14 F tract. Stones >10 mm will require fragmentation (if soft) or endoscopic sphincterotomy/surgery. Multiple stone may require repeated procedure.
7. A complete cholangiogram should be performed via the suction catheter on the day following the procedure, when the gas bubbles have cleared.

After Care

1. Pulse BP monitoring ½ hourly × 6 hours.
2. Bed rest for 12 hours.

Complication—Morbidity 4%.

Due to Contrast Medium:

1. Allergic reaction.
2. Pancreatitis.

Due to Technique:

1. Fever.
2. Perforation of T-tube tract.

Urinary Tract

Methods of Demonstration of Urinary Tract:

- Plain film including tomography.
- Excretion pyelography (I.V.P.).
- Micturating cystourethrography.
- Retrograde pyeloureterography.
- Ascending urethrography.
- Percutaneous renal puncture.
- Arteriography:
  - Aortography.
  - Selective internal iliac arteriograph for bladder.
  - Digital subtraction angiogram.
- Venography—Renal vein.
- Lymphography.
- USG.
- Radioisotope study.

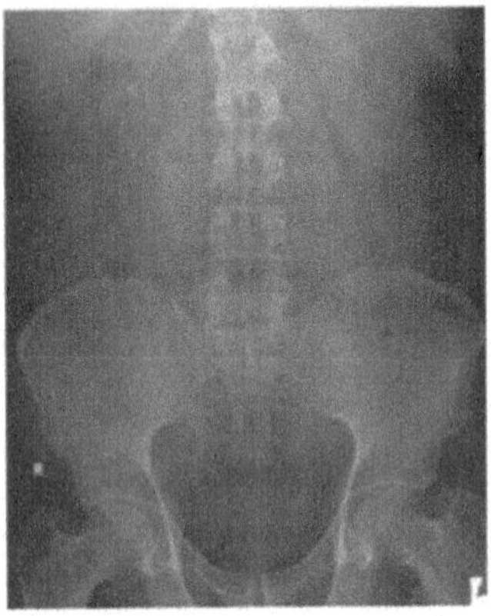

Fig. 3.19: Plain X-ray abdomen in supine position

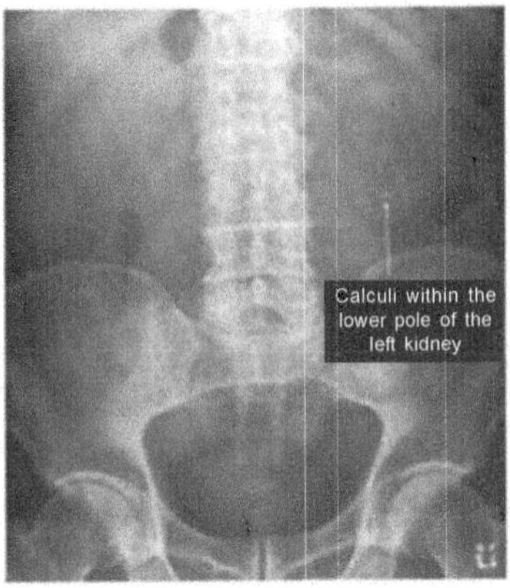

Fig. 3.20: Plain X-ray abdomen showing a kidney stone

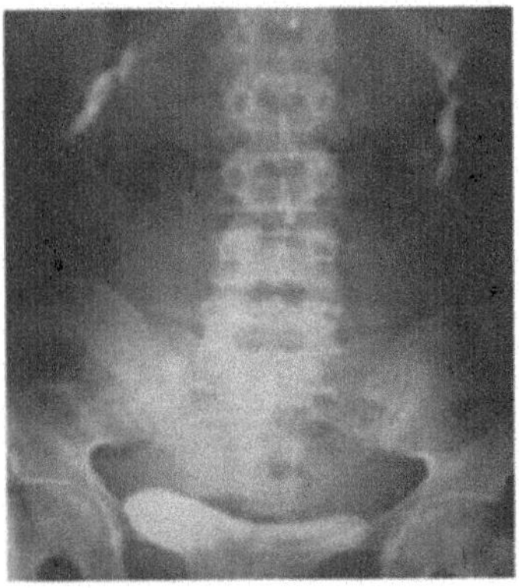

Fig. 3.21: I.V. Pyelogram showing malrotated both kidney

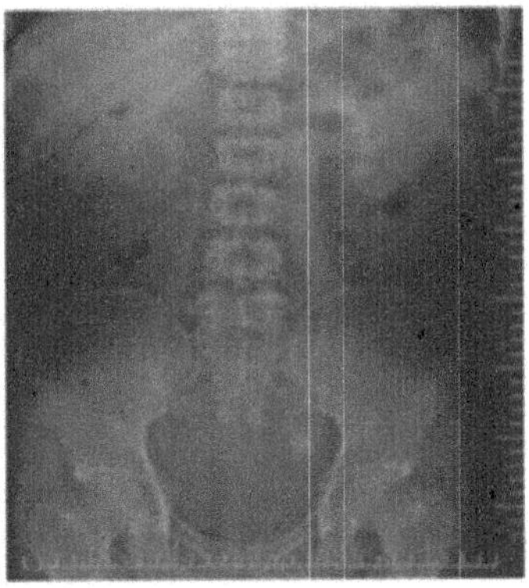

Fig. 3.22: I.V. Pyelogram: Tortuous right ureter, left hydronephroureter

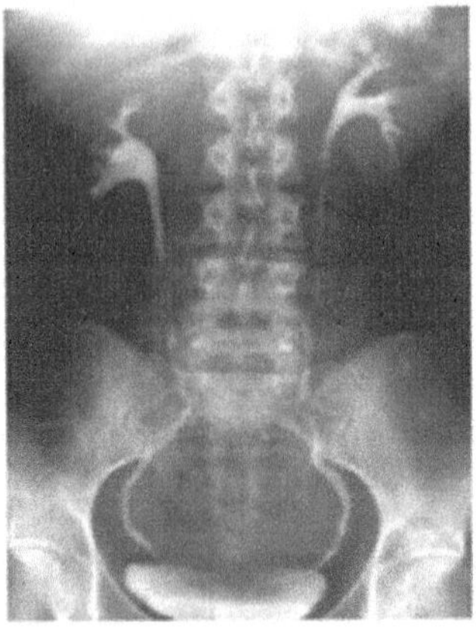

Fig. 3.23: I.V. Pyelogram: Showing both ureter in its whole length and ending into urinary bladder

- CT.
- MRI.
- Nephrotomography.
- Double contrast cystography.

I.V.P. (Excretory Urography)

This is the basic examination of urinary tract. It has the advantage of demonstrating the whole of the urinary tract.

Indication:

Suspected urinary tract pathology.

Contraindications:

1. Generalised contraindications to water soluble contrast medium.
2. Dehydration is contraindicated in following cases:
   - Renal failure (volume depletion, electrolyte imbalance deteriorating renal function).
   - Myeloma—Because of precipitation of Bence Jones protein in renal tubules.
   - Infants.

Contrast Medium:

Water soluble contrast media:

- Ionic contrast media.
- Non-ionic contrast media.

Patient's Preparations:

1. Nil orally for 5 hours prior to examination.
2. Patient should be ambulatory for 2 hours prior to exam to reduce the bowel gas.

3. Patient having earlier severe reaction to contrast media may be given prednisolone 12 hours to 4 hours prior to exam.

Preliminary Films:

1. Supine full length AP film abdomen in inspiration.
2. Supine AP of renal area in expiration.
3. 35° post oblique view.
4. Tomography of kidney.

Technique:

The median cubital vein is preferred for site of injection. A 20 gauze needle is advanced up in the vein to reduce the risk of perivenous injection and injection is given rapidly as a bolus to maximize the density of the nephrogram.

Films:

1. *Immediate film:* AP view of the renal areas (10-15 seconds after injection) for Nephrogram.
2. *5-minute film:* AP view of renal areas. To determine if excretion is symmetrical and is invaluable for assessing the need to modify the technique.

   A compression band is now applied around the patient's abdomen and the balloon positioned midway between the anterior superior iliac spine, i.e., precisely over the ureters as they cross the pelvic brim. The aim to produce better pelvicalyceal distension.

   Compression is contraindicated in:

   a. After recent abdominal surgery.
   b. After renal trauma.
   c. If there is a large abdominal mass.
   d. When the 5-minute film shows already distended calyces.
3. *15 minutes film:* AP view of renal area—There is usually adequate distension of pelvicalyceal system with opaque urine.

Compression is released when satisfactory demonstration of pelvicalyceal system has been achieved.

4. *Release film:* Supine AP abdomen. This is taken to show the whole urinary tract. If this film is satisfactory, the patient is asked to empty his bladder.
5. *After micturition film:* Coned down view of bladder with tube angled is caudad and centred 5 cm above the symphysis pubis. To demonstrate residual urine, bladder tumor, urethral diverticulum.

Additional Films:

- 35° post oblique of KUB region.
- Tomography.
- 30° caudad and angulation of the tube for renal area (to throw colon from kidneys).
- Prone abdomen—Better visualisation of ureter.
- Delayed films—In obstructive uropathy filming upto 24-48 hours.

Excretory Micturating Cystourethrography

Technique is used when further information is required regarding the urethra or the act of micturition. Excretion urography is performed in usual manner and when the bladder is full, spot films are taken of the bladder and urethra during micturition.

Complication

Due to Contrast Media.

Due to Technique: Malplaced abdominal compression may produce intolerable discomfort or hypotension.

Percutaneous Renal Puncture

Indications:

1. Renal cyst puncture.

2. Antegrade pyelography when IVP and RGP are unsuccessful and renal pressure/flow studies are required.
3. Needle nephrostomy.

Contraindications:

1. As for water soluble contrast media.
2. Bleeding diathesis.
3. Possibility of Renal Hydatid Disease.

Contrast Medium:

Water soluble contrast medium.

Equipment:

Fluoroscopic X-ray unit, over couch tube, needle, syringe.

Patient's Preparation:

1. As for excretion urography.
2. Hb, platelet count and prothrombin time.
3. Nervous patient/children need sedation.

Preliminary Film:

Supine AP view of renal areas.

Techniques:

Insertion of needle can be controlled by three methods:

1. Radiographic.
2. Using USG with/without biopsy transducer.
3. CT.

Renal Cyst Puncture

1. Kidneys are opacified by giving I.V. contrast medium.
2. The patient is then turned prone and radiolucent pad placed under the abdomen to prevent anterior movement of kidney.

Under fluoroscopic guidance site of puncture is marked on the skin.

3. Under aseptic precaution, the needle still in situ, the kidney is rescreened to note the relationship of needle to the mass.
4. Greenburg needle is introduced during suspended respiration. Needle is advanced and its position is checked by intermittent fluoroscopy. It may be deflected around the cyst and if this happens, it will be necessary to advance it into the cyst with a quick thrust.
5. The stilette is removed and the cyst content is aspirated and examined for biochemical, bacteriologically and cytologically.
6. If clear fluid is aspirated. Half the aspirated fluid is replaced with contrast media and this is repeated until the entire cyst content have been replaced with ½ of volume of contrast media. Dual contrast pictures are obtained by injecting air, less than would be needed to fill the cavity, allowing for expansion as it warms to body temperature. The needle is then removed.

Films:

Prone lateral; Rt. Lt. lateral decubitus; supine lateral; supine AP; Erect AP.

Antegrade Pyelography

The needle is introduced as far cyst is located to puncture but directed through the renal parenchyma into a minor calyx. This reduces the risk of laceration of pelvis and extravasation of urine.

Film—AP, both 35° post oblique.

Contrast media should be drained off from the distended pelvis to prevent the development of chemical pyelitis.

After Care

Chest radiograph to exclude pneumothorax.

Complication

- Due to contrast medium.
- Chemical pyelitis.
- Due to technique:
  1. Perirenal and intrarenal haemorrhage.
  2. Haematuria.
  3. Pneumothorax.
  4. Infection.
  5. Pain.
  6. Urinoma.
  7. AV fistula.
  8. Puncture of adjacent organ.

Percutaneous Nephrostomy

Introduction of a drainage catheter into the collecting system.

Indications:

1. Obstructive uropathy.
2. Ureteric fistula, internal drainage may allow closure.

Contraindication:

Uncontrolled bleeding diathesis.

Contrast Medium:

Water soluble contrast medium.

Equipment:

- 18G puncturing Longdwel needle.
- Drainage catheter—7F pigtail with multiple side holes.
- Guidewires—Conventional angiographic and Lunderquist.
- Fluoroscopy and real time USG.

Patient's Preparation:

- 4 hours fasting.
- Premedication.
- Prophylactic antibiotics.
- Surgical backup.
- Empty bladder just prior to procedure.

Technique:

- Prone or oblique position.
- Identify the collecting system by IVP, antegrade pyelography or by USG.
- A point for site of puncture in post axillary line is chosen below 12th rib.
- Skin and soft tissue are infiltrated with local anaesthetics using spinal needle.
- Puncture is made through 18G sheathed needle then J-guidewire is inserted and coiled within the collecting system. The sheath is then pushed over the wire which is exchanged for a more rigid Lunderquist wire. If possible guidewire is manipulated into the ureter. Dilatation is then performed to 1F greater than the size of drainage catheter, which is then inserted. During the procedure, care must be taken that guidewire is not kinked into the soft tissue. A substantial amount of guidewire should be maintained within the collecting system so that position is not lost and if kinking does occur then kinked portion of the wire can be withdrawn outside the skin.
- Cope needle system—Using a 21G puncturing needle that takes a special guidewire. This affords a single puncture with a fine needle, leading on to eventual catheterization.
- Trocar cannula system—In which direct puncture of collecting system is made with the drainage catheter already assembled

over a trocar. On removal of the trocar, the drainage catheter is pushed further into the collecting system.

Having successfully introduced a catheter, the latter is securely fixed to the skin and drainage commenced.

After Care

- Bed rest for 12 hours.
- BP temp ½ hourly × 6 hours.
- Urine C/s.

Complications

1. Unsuccessful drainage.
2. Haemorrhage.
3. Perforation of collecting system.
4. Septicaemia.

Retrograde Pyelogram

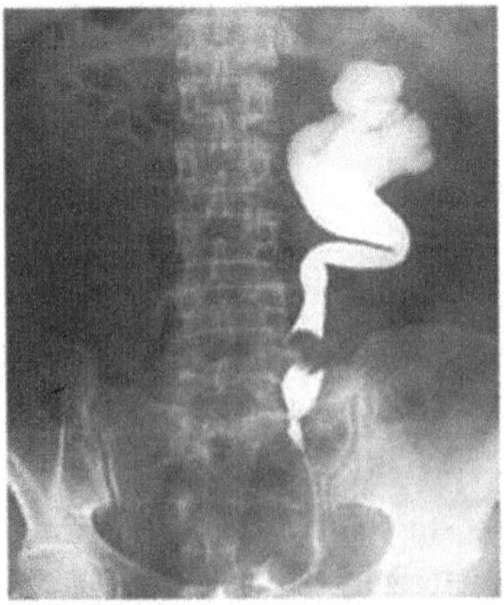

Fig. 3.24: Retrograde pyelogram: Showing a radiolucent calculus in left ureter causing hydronephrosis

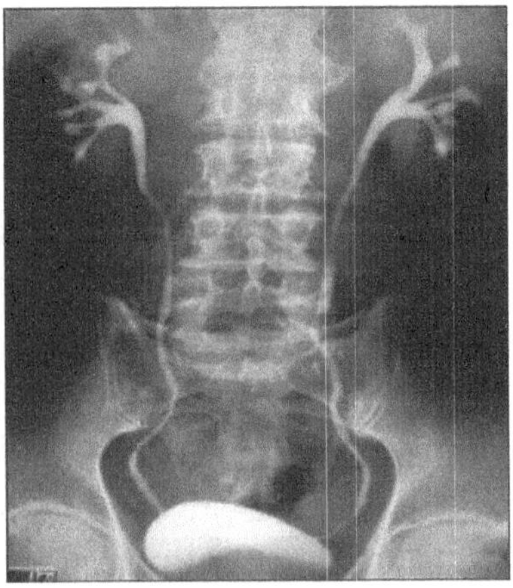

Fig. 3.25: Bilateral retrograde pyelogram

Indication:

1. To demonstrate pelvicalyceal system after an unsatisfactory excretory pyelogram.
2. To demonstrate the site, length, lower limit if possible nature of an obstructive lesion.

Contraindications:

Acute urinary tract infection.

Contrast Medium:

Water soluble contrast medium.

Equipment:

1. Fluoroscopy X-ray unit with spot film device.
2. Ureteral catheter.

Patient Preparation:

G.A./epidural.

Preliminary Film:

K.U.B. abdomen skiagram.

Technique:

1. With ureteral catheter in situ, the patient is transferred from O.T. to X-ray department.
2. Urine is evacuated and under fluoroscopic control contrast medium is slowly injected. About 5 ml are enough to fill the pelvis however the injection should be terminated if the patient complains of pain or fullness in loin. Supine PA view of kidney and bilat. 35° ant. oblique films of kidneys are obtained.
3. If there is pelvic ureteric function obstruction, the contrast medium in the pelvis is aspirated. If the exam is satisfactory, the catheter is withdrawn, first to 10 cm below the renal pelvis and then to lie just above the ureteric orifice.

About 2 ml of contrast medium are injected at each of these level and films are taken.

After Care

1. Post anesthetic observation.
2. Prophylactic antibiotic.

Complication

As in GA.

Due to Contrast Medium—After absorption from renal pelvis, adverse reaction may take place.

- Chemical pyelitis.
- Extravasation due to overdistension of pelvis.

Due to Techniques:

- Infection.
- Mucosal damage of water.
- Perforation of ureter or pelvis by catheter.

Micturating Cystourethrogram

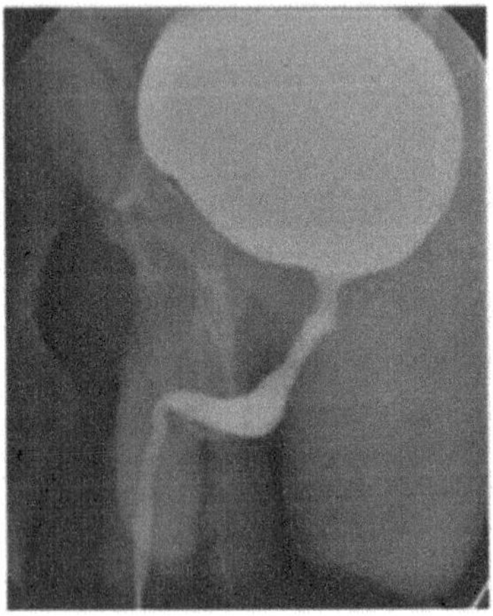

Fig. 3.26: Micturating cystourethrogram

Indications:

1. Vesicoureteral reflux.
2. Study of urethra during micturition.
3. Abnormalities of bladder.
4. Stress incontinence.

Contraindications:

Acute U.T.I.

Contrast Medium:

Water soluble contrast medium.

Equipment:

1. Fluoroscopy X-ray unit with spot film device.
2. Video recorder.
3. Foley's catheter.

Patient Preparation:

Evacuate the bladder before examination.

Preliminary Film:

Coned view of bladder.

Technique:

VUR—Patient lies supine on X-ray table, using aseptic technique, a catheter lubricated with glycerine is introduced into the bladder. Residual urine is drained. Contrast medium is slowly dripped into bladder filling is observed by intermittent fluoroscopy.

Any reflux is recorded on spot film.

Then micturition is processed and when the patient is micturating in oblique position, so that full length of urethra is visualised.

This view also demonstrate VUR.

For demonstration of stress incontinence; the film should include sacrum and symphysis pubis because the bony landmarks are used to assess the bladder neck descent.

1. Lateral bladder.
2. Lateral bladder straining.

   Then the catheter is removed.

3. Lateral bladder during micturition.

After Care

Dysuria—analgesic.

Complications

Due to Contrast Media—Chemical cystitis.

Due to technique—Acute UTI, catheter trauma, perforation due to over distension, retention of Foley catheter and catheterization of vagina or an ectopic ureteral orifice.

Ascending Urethrography in Male

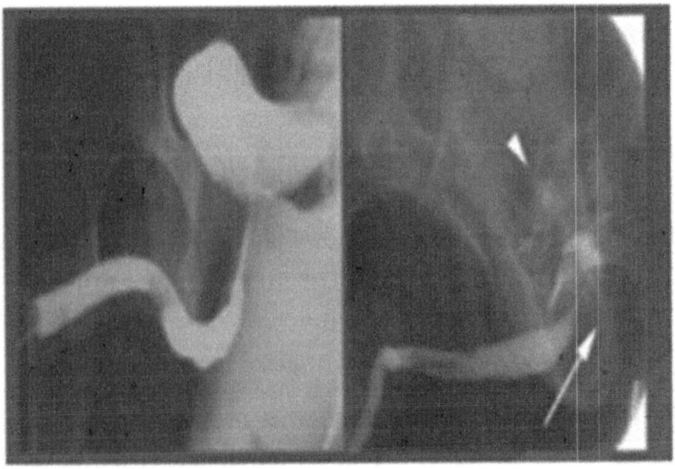

Fig. 3.27: Retrograde urethrogram

Indications:

- Stricture.
- Urethral tear.
- Cong. abnormalities.
- Periurethral or prostatic abscess.
- Fistulae or false passage.

Contraindications:

- Acute UTI.
- Recent instrumentation.

Contrast Medium:

Water soluble contrast medium.

Equipment:

- Fluoroscopy X-ray unit with spot film device.
- Penile clamp Knutsson's or Foley catheter.

Patient Preparation:

None.

Preliminary Film:

Coned view of bladder base and urethra.

Technique:

Foley catheter is introduced into urethra after lubricating it with xylocain creme. Balloon is inflated with 1-2 ml of water. The balloon lie in fossa navicularis. Water soluble contrast media is injected under fluoroscopic control and films are taken:

1. 30° LAO with right leg abducted and knee flexed.
2. Supine PA.
3. 30° RAO with left leg abducted and knee flexed.

It should be followed by micturating cystourethrogram to demonstrate the proximal urethra. Occasionally a urethral fistula or periurethral abscess is seen only on voiding film. Reflux of contrast medium into dilated prostatic ducts is better seen during micturition.

After Care:

None.

Complication

Due to Contrast Media.

Due to Technique—Acute, UTI, urethral trauma, extravasation of contrast media especially if excessive pressure is used to overcome a stricture.

Percutaneous Nephrolithotomy

Removal of renal calculi through a nephrostomy tract.

Indications:

1. Removal of renal stone.
2. Disintegration of large renal calculi.

Contraindication:

Uncontrolled bleeding diathesis.

Contrast Medium:

Water soluble contrast medium.

Equipment:

- 18G puncturing needle "Longdwel".
- Guidewire including J-angiographic and Lunderquist.
- Tract dilating equipment, Teflon dilators (7°F-30°F) metal coaxial dilators or special angioplasty balloon catheter.
- Fluoroscopy facilities with rotating C-arm.

Patient Preparation:

- Full discussion between radiologist/urologist concerning indications.
- Admission on the day prior to the procedure. G.A. is required.
- Coagulation screen.
- Two units of blood crossmatched.
- Antibiotic.
- Premedication.
- Bladder catheterization.

Technique:

IVP is done to opacify the collecting system. Retrograde ureteric catheterization, distension of collecting system is achieved. Antegrade pyelography enables distension of collecting system. A lower pole posterior calyx is chosen if the calculus is stimulated in the renal pelvis. Otherwise the calyx in which the calculus is situated must be punctured. Special care must be taken if puncturing above 12th rib because of risk of perforating the diaphragm and pleura. Puncture is in an oblique plane from post axillary line through the renal parenchyma. Puncture of the selected calyx is made using either a rotating C-arm fluoroscopy or rocking the patient to determine the depth of the calyx in relation to needle tip. On successful puncture a J-guidewire is inserted through the sheath and as much wire as possible is guided into collecting system. The sheath is then pushed over the wire, which is exchanged for a more rigid Lunderquist wire. If possible the wire is manipulated into the ureter. At this stage full dilatation may be performed or a nephrostomy tube left in situ with dilatation later.

This is carried out under GA. It is performed using Teflon dilators from 7°F to 30°F which are introduced over a guidewire. Alternatively metal coaxial dilators or a special angioplasty balloon (10 cm long) are used. A sheath is inserted over the largest dilator or balloon and through the sheath lumen removal of calculus or disintegration is performed.

Removal of calculi of less than 1 cm is possible with use of a nephroscope and forceps. Larger calculi must be disintegrated using an ultrasonic or electrohydraulic disintegrator.

After Care

- Usually determined by anesthetist/urologist.
- Plain X-ray of kidney region to ensure that all calculi fragments have been removed.

Complications

Immediate:

- Failure of access, dilatation or removal.
- Perforation of renal pelvis on dilatation.
- Haemorrhage.
- Damage to surrounding structure, i.e., diaphragm, colon, spleen and liver.
- Problems related to irrigating fluid, i.e., haemolysis.

Delayed:

Aneurysm of an intrarenal artery.

Reproductive System

Methods to demonstrate female reproductive system:

1. Plain abdomen.
2. HSG (Hysterosalpingogram).
3. Gynaecography.
4. Arteriography.
5. Lymphography.
6. USG.

7. CT.
8. MRI.

Hysterosalpingography

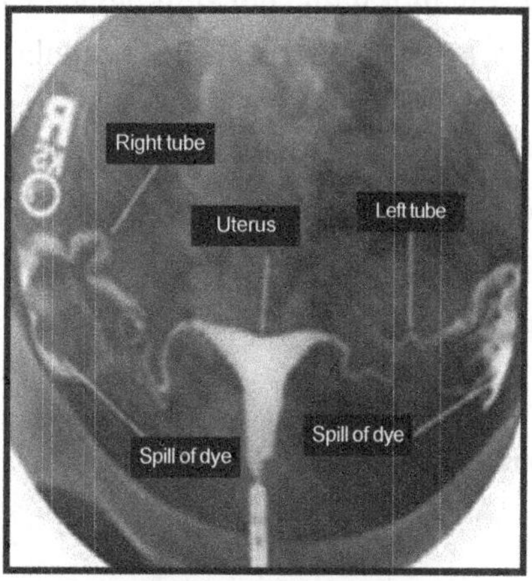

Fig. 3.28: Hysterosalpingogram

Indication:

- Infertility.
- Recurrent abortion.
- Following tubal surgery.

Contraindications:

- Pregnancy.
- A purulent discharge on inspection of the vulva/cervix.
- Recurrent dilatation and curettage or abortion or immediately post-menstruation.

Contrast Medium:

Water soluble contrast medium.

Advantage:

Rapid peritoneal spill ensures and short procedure time.

Disadvantage:

Peritoneal spill is more painful.

Equipment:

Fluoroscopic X-ray unit with spot film device vaginal speculum, vulsellum forcep, uterine sound and HSG canula.

Patient Preparation:

1. Examination should be done between 5th and10th day of menstrual cycle.
2. Premedication:
   - Diazepam.
   - Buscopan.

Technique:

Patient lies supine on table with knees flexed, legs abducted and heels together under aseptic atmosphere, gynaecologist inserts a speculum and cleans the vagina and cervix with chlorhexidine. Anterior lip of cervix is steadied with vulsellum forceps and canula is inserted into cervical canal after assessment of uterine cavity with the help of uterine sound. Care must be taken to expel all air bubbles from syringe and canula as these would otherwise cause confusion in interpretation. Contrast medium is injected slowly under intermittent fluoroscopic control. Three films are taken to demonstrate the peritoneal spillage.

Instruments are taken out and cotton pad is given for any soakage after investigation.

After Care

She must be advised that there may be bleeding per vagina for 1-2 days and analgesic and antibiotic are given.

Complications

- Idiosyncrasy.
- Oil granuloma.
- Oil emboli.

Due to Technique:

1. Pain—While using vulsellem forcep during insertion of canula with tubal distension proximal to site of block with distension of uterus if there is tubal spasm with peritoneal irritation during following week.
2. Bleeding from trauma to uterus or cervix.
3. Infection.
4. Abortion.

Gynaecography

Indications:

Ovarian pathology, especially Stein-Leventhal syndrome and ovarian agenesis.

Nowadays it is not done and USG is investigation of choice.

Vesiculography

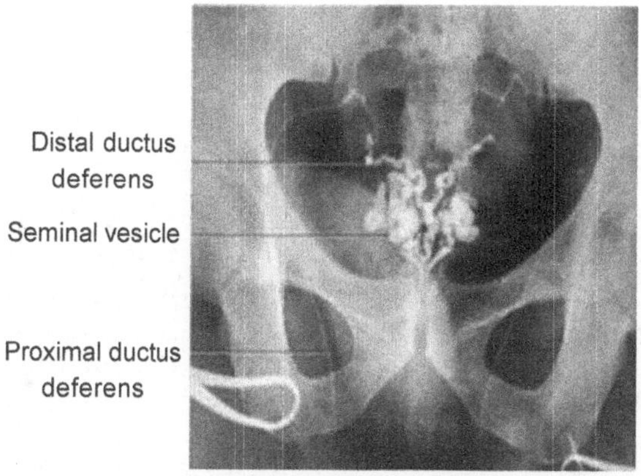

Fig. 3.29: Vesiculogram

Methods:

- Vaso-seminal route.
- Transurethral route.

Indications:

1. Ill defined pain in testis, perineum or coccygeal region, which may be due to seminal tract disease.
2. Patency of vasa after repair of vasectomy.
3. Sterility.
4. Staging of prostatic carcinoma.

Contraindications: None.

Technique: Acute epididymoorchitis technique, under aseptic precaution the vas deferens is isolated 4 cm below the inguinal ring. The skin is infiltrated with Lignocain and incised, the vas is brought out through the opening and separated from its fascial covering. The vas is cannulated using a 25 G butterfly needle. The procedure is repeated on the opposite side, contrast medium is slowly injected on both sides simultaneously.

Transurethral route: The ejaculatory ducts may be catheterized at their opening on the verumontanum using a special urethroscope.

Respiratory System

Methods of demonstration of respiratory system:

1. Plain films.
2. Tomography.
3. Xero radiography.
4. Nasopharyngography.
5. Laryngography.
6. Tracheography.

7. Bronchography.
8. Radioisotope study:
   - Ventilation 8^{1m}k or ^{133}xe.
   - Perfusion—^{99m}Tc microsphere of human albumin.
9. CT.
10. MRI.
11. USG.

All these techniques except USG, CT and MRI are now abandoned.

Arteriography and Angiocardiography

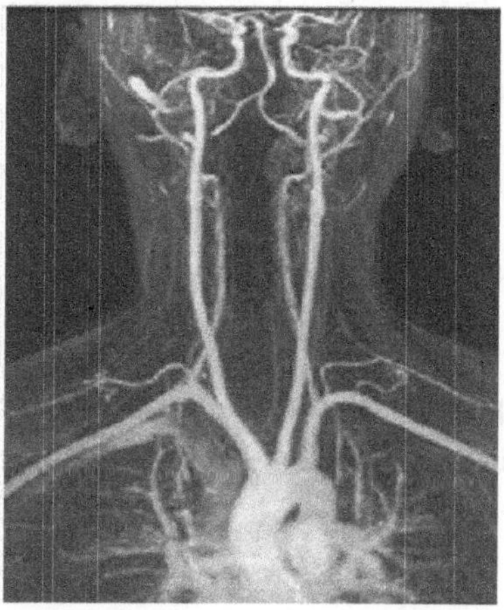

Fig. 3.30: Arteriogram showing arch of aorta, its branches in the neck

Methods of demonstration of heart and great vessels:

1. Chest radiograph—PA, Penetrated PA, Left lateral, Left oblique.
2. Barium swallow in RAO position to assess left atrial enlargement.
3. Fluoroscopy.
4. Tomography.

5. Angiocardiography.
6. Aortography.
7. Superior and inferior vena cavography.
8. Pulmonary arteriography.
9. Echocardiography:
   - M-mode.
   - 2-D.
   - Doppler study.
10. Radioisotope:

    Myocardial perfusion imaging with 201 Thallium radionuclide ventriculography using ^{99m}Tc labelled RBC or human serum albumin.
11. CT.
12. MRI.

Equipments for an Angiography Room

X-ray generator—3 phase, 12 pulse and at least 1000 mA. For biplane angiography of 1000 mA generators are better than one 2000 mA generator because:

1. A fault in one generator will not put all the X-ray apparatus out of action.
2. Completely different exposure values can be set for AP and lateral views.

X-ray Tube—High speed, rotating anode with 0.6 mm^2 focal spot. Two tubes will be needed for biplane angiography and are essential for investigating congenital heart disease. A 0.3 mm^2 focal spot is necessary for macroangiography. A C- or U arm device in which X-ray tube and intensifier are placed at opposite ends of a C-arm or U-shaped frame which can be rotated round the patient has number of advantages:

1. Patient does not need to be disturbed during the procedure.
2. There is less likelihood of dislodgement of catheter.
3. Axial view.

Disadvantages:

- More space is required.
- Expensive.

Fluoroscopy and cine radiography, videorecorder, rapid serial film changer, pressure injector, pressure monitoring equipment, ECG monitor, resuscitation equipment.

Introduction to Catheter Technique

The basic technique of arterial catheterization is applicable to veins also.

Patient Preparation:

1. Hospitalisation of patient for 24 hours observation before and after the investigation.
2. Discontinue anticoagulants.
3. Patient is explained about procedure. Consent is obtained. Examine the patient for BP, peripheral pulse.
4. Puncture site is shaved.
5. Premedication.

Puncture Site:

- Femoral artery.
- Axillary artery.
- Brachial artery.
- Aorta.

Types of Angiogram

- Head and neck arteriography.

- Angiocardiography.
- Pulmonary arteriography.
- Coronary arteriography.
- Ascending aortography.
- Translumbar aortography.
- Arteriography of lower limb.
- Coeliac axis, superior mesenteric and inferiormesenteric anteriography.
- Renal arteriography.

All these techniques are replaced with color doppler sonography, 3-D multisliced CT and MR angiography.

Venography

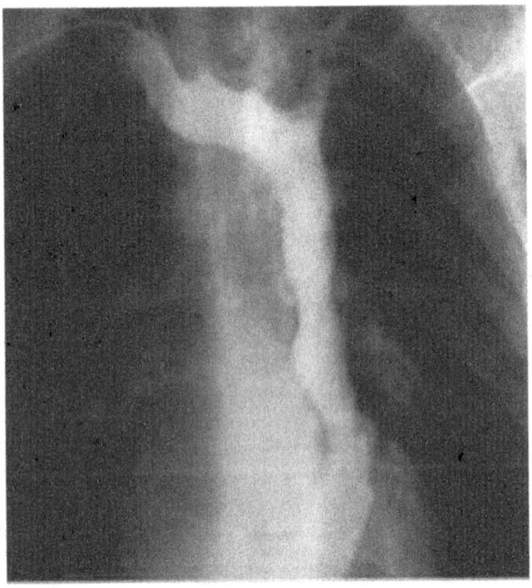

Fig. 3.31: Venogram showing superior vena cava and azygos vein

Method of demonstration of venous system:

- Contrast medium venography:
  - I.V.
  - Interosseous.

- USG.
- Radioisotope study:
  - ^{125}I fibrinogen
  - ^{99m}Tc macro aggregates
  - ^{99m}Tc plasmin
  - ^{99m}Tc urokinase
  - ^{99m}Tc in platelets.
- Peripheral venography:
  - Lower limb.
  - Upper limb.
- Superior vena cavography.
- Inferior vena cavography.
- Pelvic venography.
- Ascending lumbar venography.
- Intraosseous venography.
- Portal venography.
- Transhepatic portal venous catheterization.
- Selective retrograde venography.
- Hepatic venography.
- Internal jugular venography.
- Orbital venography.

All these techniques have been replaced by color doppler sonography, multisliced CT scan and MR venographic techniques.

Lymph Gland and Lymphatics

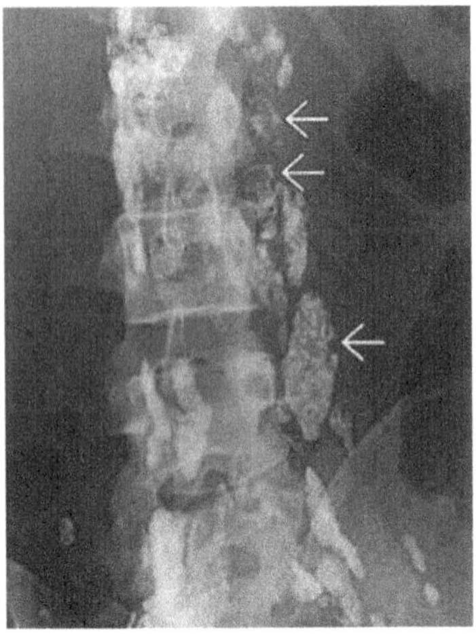

Fig. 3.32: Lymphangiogram showing lymphatics

Methods of Demonstration of Lymph Glands:

a. Plain film may show:
   1. A soft tissue mass, hilar lymph node.
   2. Calcification—Mesenteric glands and tubercular glands in pulmonary hila.

b. Indirect evidence from displacement of normal structure, e.g., displacement of ureters seen during IVP or displacement of IVC during IV cavography.

c. Lymphography:

   Advantage:
   1. Can detect tumor within normal sized LN.
   2. Can distinguish reactive LN from tumor containing LN.
   3. Enables surveillance of residually opacified glands over several months.

   Disadvantage:
   1. Does not image internal iliac, mesenteric, retrocrural, splenic and renal hilar nodes.

2. Liver and spleen are not visualised.
3. Uncomfortable and technical skill needed for cannulation.

d. CT:

Advantage:

1. Can image all intra-abdominal glands.
2. Technically easier to perform.

Disadvantage:

1. Not widely available.
2. Internal structure of gland is not seen.
3. Retroperitoneal glands are difficult to define if there is paucity of retroperitoneal fat.

e. USG:

Advantage:

1. Non-invasive and without risk to patient.

Disadvantage:

1. Highly operator dependent.
2. Intestinal gas is a major factor in poor visualization.
3. The internal structure of LN is not seen.

f. Radioisotope study:

1. 67 gallium citrate—Hodgkin's lymphoma.
2. ^{99m}Tc—antimony colloid and ^{99m}Tc-sulphur colloid injected subcutancously into the medial web of each foot and after gentle exercise. The pelvis and abdomen are imaged during next 90-150 minutes.
3. Internal mammary lymphoscintigraphy—using ^{99m}Tc antimony colloid injected into posterior rectus sheath.

Arthrography

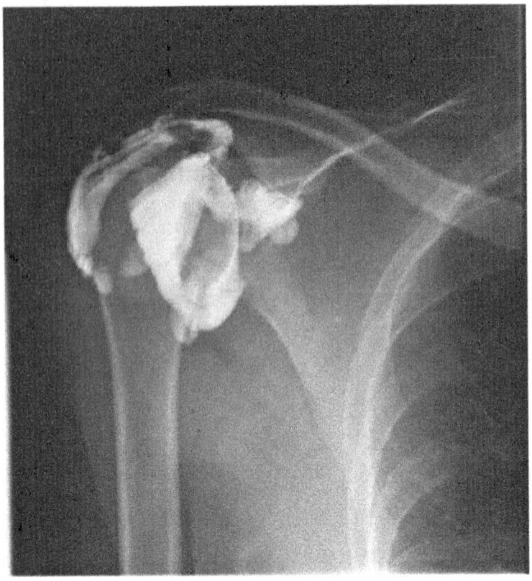

Fig. 3.33: Arthrography of shoulder joint

- Double contrast knee arthrography.
- Hip arthrography.
- Double contrast shoulder arthrography.
- Elbow arthrography.
- Wrist arthrography.
- Ankle arthrography.
- TMJ arthrography.

Replaced by MRI.

Central Nervous System

Methods of Demonstration of Brain:

- Plain film.
- Tomography.
- Angiography.

- Air encephalography.
- Ventriculography.
- Cisternography.
- CT.
- Radioisotope.
- USG.
- MRI.
- PET.
- PET-CT.

Methods of Demonstration of Spinal Canal:

- Plain film.
- Tomogram.
- Myelogram.
- Discogram.
- Epidurogram.
- Ascending lumbar venography.
- CT.
- USG.
- Arteriography.
- MRI.
- Best way to demonstrate spinal canal is MRI.

Dacryocystography

Indication:

Epiphora, to demonstrate the site and degree of obstruction.

Sialography

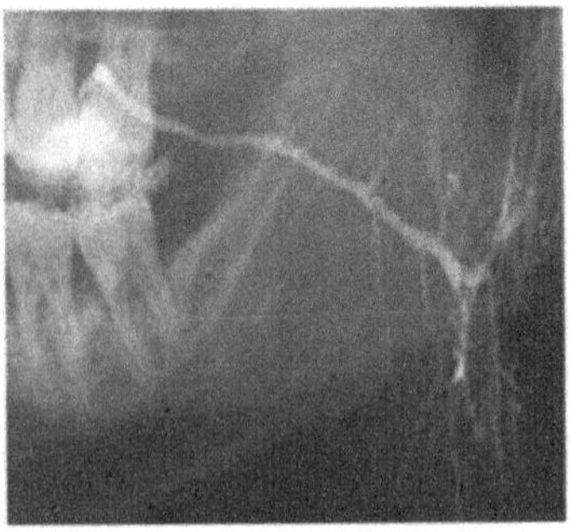

Fig. 3.34: Parotid sialography

Indication:

Pain and recurrent swelling.

Contraindication:

Acute infection on inflammation.

Contrast Medium:

Water soluble contrast.

Equipment:

Skull unit, silver lacrimal dilator, silver cannula or 18G blunt needle and polyethylene catheter.

Patient Preparation:

Remove opaque artefact.

Preliminary Film:

AP with head rotated 5° away from the side of exam with centre to the midline of lower lip.

Parotid Gland:

- Lateral view—centre to angle of mandible.
- Lateral oblique view—centre to angle of mandible and with tube angled 20° cephalad.

Submandibular Gland

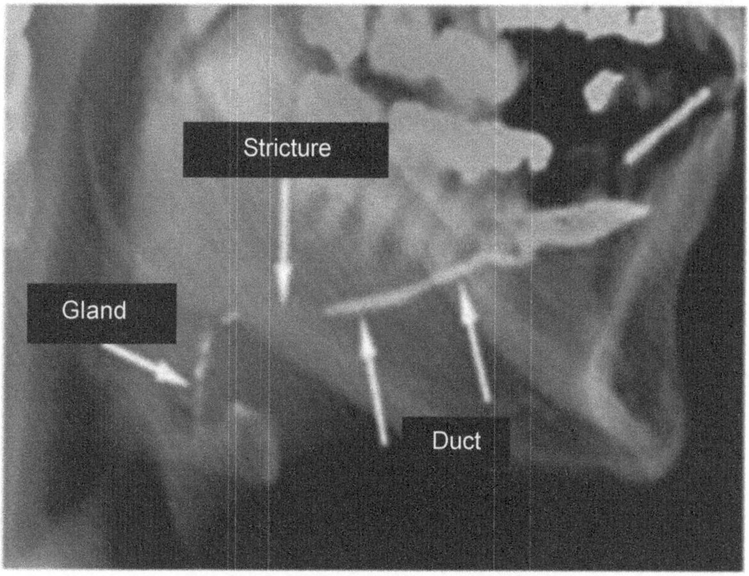

Fig. 3.35: Submandibular sialography

- Inferosuperior view—using occlusal film.
- Lateral view with floor of mouth depressed by a wooden spatula.
- Lateral oblique view—centre 1 cm anterior to the angle of mandible, tube angled 20° cephalad.

Technique:

Orifice of parotid duct is adjacent to crown of 2nd upper molar and that of submandibular duct is at the base of frenulum of tongue. If they are not visible, lemon juice is placed in mouth to promote secretion of gland, so render the orifice visible.

Orifice of duct is dilated with silver wire probe and cannula or polythene catheter is introduced into the duct.

2 cc of contrast media is injected. The duct must not be overfilled. If pain—no further injection of contrast medium.

Film:

- Immediate.
- Post secretory.

After Care:

None.

Complication

Pain, damage to duct orifice, rupture of duct infection.

4
Ultrasonography

TECHNICAL ASPECT

Characteristics of Ultrasound

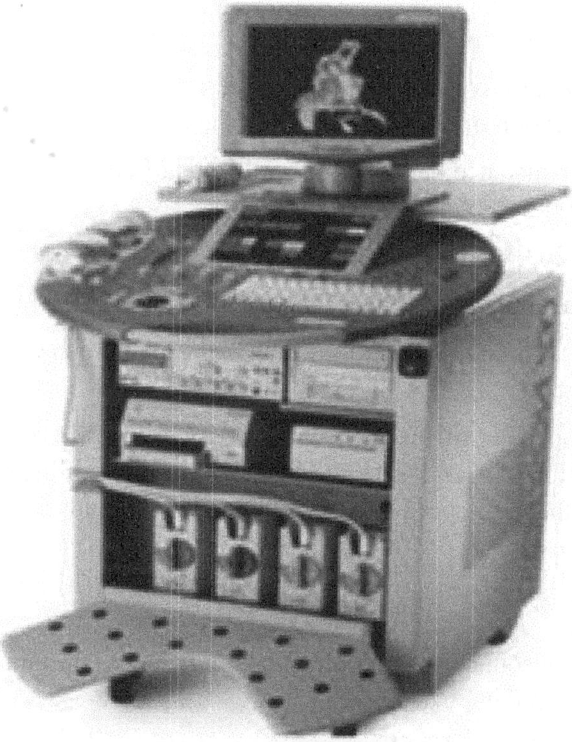

Fig. 4.1: Ultrasound machine

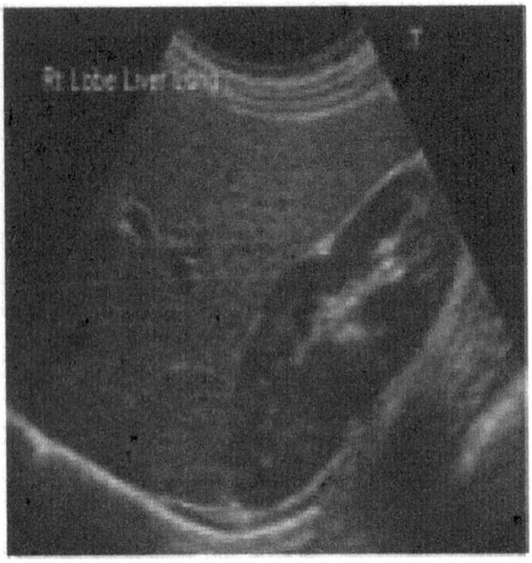

Fig. 4.2: Ultrasonography of liver, right kidney also seen

1. Sound wave transmitting energy.
2. Require a medium for transmission.
3. Longitudinal waves, i.e., particles of the medium move parallel to the direction of propagation of the wave.
4. λ = is the distance between the two bands of compression of rarefaction.
5. ν = is > 20,000 Hz.

   In clinical application, it is in the range of 2-50 MHz.
6. Velocity of sound changes according to the medium in which it traverses.

   Two properties of the medium contribute in affecting the propagation of sound through (either by compressibility or by density) them. So speed is more in solid, then in liquids followed less in gases.

   $$\text{Equation: } V = \nu\lambda$$

   Velocity of sound in a particular medium remains constant so if ν increased then λ decreases.
7. Intensity of sound/Loudness.

   High intensity—compression bands are more compacted.

Intensity of sound decreases and not the v. expressed in decibels.

Transducers

It is defined as an assembly or device that converts one form of energy into another, i.e., they convert an electric signal into ultrasonic energy that is transmitted to the tissues and ultrasonic energy reflected back from the tissue into electronic signals.

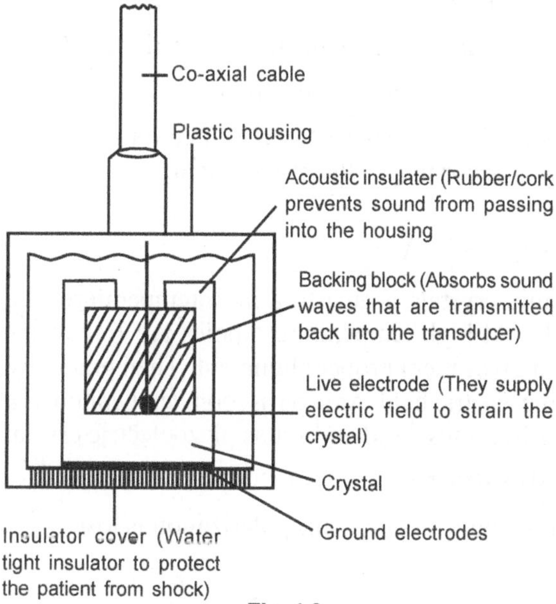

Fig. 4.3

Backing block is tungsten or rubber powder in an epoxy resin ratio of tungsten/resin-satisfies impedance requirement. Rubber increases the attenuation of sound in this block.

Piezoelectric Crystals

Most important component. This principle was discovered by Pierre Curie in 1880.

They have the unique property to change shape when electric field is applied across them and also when sound waves reflected from the body to reach the transducer.

It causes physical compression of the crystal element. This forces the tiny dipoles to change their orientation and thus induces the voltage, called as "Pressure Electricity".

Crystal used are:

Natural : Quartz.

Artificial : Called as ferroelectric (Ceramics), e.g., Barium titanate (used for first time) Lead Zirconate Titanate (PZT).

Many others with slight alterations in PZT.

New—Ferroelectric relaxors.

Advantages : These crystals can be formed into different shapes according to the requirement.

How to Prepare?

These ceramic crystals heated to a high temperature in a strong electric field. At high temperature dipoles are free to move and electric field gives them proper alignment. Then gradually cooled keeping in the electric field. As soon as room temperature is attained, then dipoles becomes fixed and act as piezoelectric crystal.

Curie Temperature

It is the temperature at which this polarization is lost.

Properties:

1. Crystals have a characteristic resonant frequency. Thickness of the crystal determines its natural ν. When crystal is struck with a voltage, it vibrates at its natural ν which is one that produces λ that are twice the thickness of the crystal.

$$\lambda = 2t$$

$$\frac{t}{\lambda} = 2t$$

$$\nu = \frac{V}{X}$$

X: In medical ultrasound, the transducer is drawn at its resonant ν.

2. Transducer Q factors:

It refer to two properties of piezoelectric crystal.

- Purity of their sound.
- Length of time that the sound persists.

Ring down time—Is time between the initiation of the wave and complete cessation of librations is called the ring down time.

Pulse length—The length of the sonic pulse = number of waves × wavelength.

Crystals with:

High Q : Narrow ν range

: High ring down time hence high pulse length.

Low Q : Wide ν spectrum

: Low ring down time.

Q Factor : Can be varied by altering the character of backing block. It quenches the vibration and shortens the sonic pulse.

In medical imaging transducers are pulsed for 2-3 cycles only.

3. Acoustic impedance (Z) = 8 c–of the backing block so that the sound directed away from the patient will be transmitted into and absorbed by the backing block.
4. Mineral oil/any coupling material is applied between the patient skin and transducer, for effective transmission of energy from the transducer to the patient. Coupling needed to prevent any air gap or contact scanning.

5. Matching layer—It is a method of improving energy transfer by mechanical impedance matching with suitable thickness and characteristic impedance placed on the front of the transducer so that energy is transmitted to patient effectively.

Types of Transducer

Array Transducer

Having an array of small crystals.

- Linear.
- Phased.
- Curved.
- Annular.

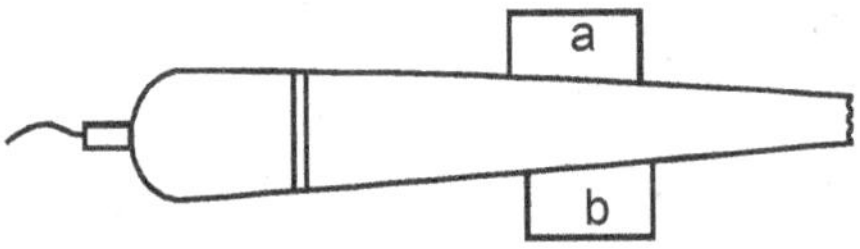

Focussed Transducer

1. Improve lateral resolution.
2. They restrict beam width but they are designed to focus a specific depth/depth range.

Focussing done with:

- Curved piezoelectric crystal
- Acoustic lens → Polystyrene / Epoxy resin
  - These propagate sound at greater velocity so beam is refracted and bent towards a point in space where greatest intensity beam is seen, i.e., called as focal point or rather focal zone.
- *Electronically*—Focal position can be altered by changing the delays within the transmitted pulse, i.e., dynamic focussing.

Thickness = ¼ λ of sound in matching layer hence termed as Quarter wave matching.

So typical transducer compress from the surface. It has various layers:

1. Protective layer.
2. Acoustic lens.
3. Matching layer.
4. PZT.
5. Backing block.

Modes

M-Mode (Movement Mode): In 'A' mode, the echoes are produced by moving structures then the echo spikes will also move with time. Here the spikes are replaced by dots and movement of dots are plotted with time → TM mode (Time-Motion study).

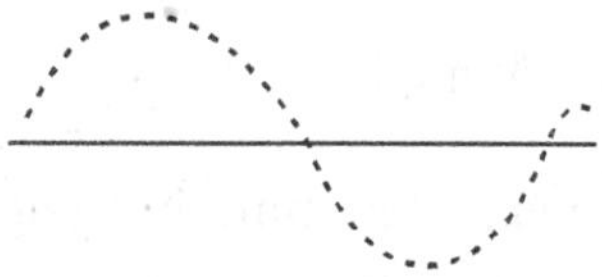

Used for electrocardiography.

B-Mode (Brightness Mode): It provides two-dimensional tomographic image of the body, formed by sweeping of the beam a slice of tissue and mapping the echogenicity of the reflectors as shades of grey to for β-mode scan or grey scale scan.

Digital scan converter tubes used now for:

- Good memory.
- Better resolution.
- Data processing.

Depth determined by pulse-echo principle and lateral position is determined by the direction in which beam was sent.

Ultrasonic Display: Ultrasonic images—It is an electric representation of data generated from returning echoes and displayed on a TV monitor.

Pulse-Echo Method: Signals are displayed corresponding to the depth calculated from the time elapsed between transmission and receipt of the echos.

A-Mode (Amplitude Mode)

(Single dimension)

Echo intensity

depth

Baseline identifies the central axis of the beam.

1. Depth of the echo producing interface is determined. The depth of the interface is determined according to the time, it takes for the echoes to return.
2. Strength/amplitude of the echo is determined by the height of reflection.

Used in – Ophthalmology.

– Echoencephalography.

Real Time Ultrasound: Real time imaging system are those that have frame rates fast enough to allow movement to be followed.

B-mode system produces a single image frame.

Mechanical Transducer

Used as simple single or 2-3 element which is mechanically swept through the arc (typically by 360°) by spinning it. Resulting image has a circular shape with transducer at the centre. Used now only for—intravascular ultrasound and TRUS.

If array of crystals used—called as annular array.

Basic principle is—a piece of crystal is replaced by numerous small units each with its own electrodes.

Each ~ 1 mm in width and 5-10 mm in length.

Electronic Transducer

2 types — Linear
— Phased/sector array

Linear: Produces rectangular scan format. Individual elements are arranged in linear fashion. Beam is moved across the scanned plane by firing the elements in groups starting from one end of the array.

Used for superficial structure, small parts, vascular and obstetrics.

Curved Array: It is a variety of linear array. They are shaped as a curve convex. So that FOV is trapezoidal. They provide large FOV with sector transducer.

Useful for both superficial and deeper structure.

Use for obstetric, in TVS and TRUS probes, pediatric imaging.

Sector System/Phased Array/Steered Array: A sector scan is obtained. Each crystal has separate electrical contacts and pulses to each element are serially delayed from one end of the array to the other. These minute differences occur within short time needed to form an individual pulse, thus produce an interference pattern in between troughs and peak if pressure waves and where they coincide and subtract, they are out of phase (hence phased arrays). It results in a beam that is directed away from the straight ahead direction. For the next set slightly different set of delays is applied for beam stearin. Advantage—it allows small skin contact, though poor superficial resolution.

Newer Developments in USG

1. High v probes
   - Fast microprocessors.
   - Automatic TGC.
   - Reduce speckle.
   - Clutter suppression.

2. 3D.
3. 4D.
4. Elastography.
5. Contrast agents.
6. Contrast specific imaging.

3D USG: It allows the simultaneous assessment of individual in sectional planes. Also allows demonstration of the coronal plane and to the transducer face facilitating the identification of surface irregularities.

It helps to assess volume estimation. For this two methods are available:

1. Conventional full planner or contour method.
2. Rotational method—Possible through VOCAL imaging programme.

   VOCAL = Virtual organ computer aided analysis.

VOCAL method facilitates assessment of blood flow in a novel manner by Quantification of the power Doppler signal in the defined volume of interest and within the surrounding tissue.

Three indices of vascularity are calculated:

1. Vascularization index (VI).
2. Flow index.
3. Vascularization flow index.

It allows better assessment of:

1. Uterine anomalies.
2. Intrauterine pathology.
3. Polycystic ovaries.
4. Endometriosis.
5. Ovarian torsion.
6. 3D markers of ovarian reserve, endometrial receptivity.

Image Quality

- Spatial resolution.
- Contrast resolution.
- Temporal resolution.
- Free from artefact.

Spatial Resolution: Ability to differentiate, closely spaced objects as two district entities estimated in all the 3 dimensions.

a. *Axial/Depth Resolution:*

- Along the axis of the beam.
- It is determined by pulse length.
- Two objects will be resolved if the spatial pulse length is less than twice the separation.
- Higher the $\nu \rightarrow \downarrow$ the $\lambda \rightarrow \downarrow$ the pulse length $\rightarrow$ Higher the resolution.
- Can be kept short by using a backing block and shortening electronic shock. Usually emitted pulse with N 2 λ long.

b. *Lateral Resolution:*

- Ability to separate two adjacent objects, i.e., in a plane vertical to the beam and parallel to the transducer.
- To recognize the objects as discreter entities, beam must be narrower than the space separating the objects.
- It can be achieved in 2 ways:
  - Use of lenses:
    - Electrical.
    - Mechanical.
  - Use of large aperture transducers.

c. *Azimuth/Elevation Resolution:* Refers to slice thickness in a plane vertical to both beam and transducer.

Character of US Beam

1. It forms concentric ring with together at some distance from a wavefront.
2. Intensity of sound—decreases with distance.

Major drawback—poor penetration, as tissue absorption increases with ν.

Interactions Between US and Matter

- Reflection.
- Refraction.
- Attenuation.

1. **Reflection**—Image is produced by the reflected beam. The percentage of beam reflected at tissue interfaces depends upon:
   - Tissues acoustic impedance.
   - Beams of incidence.

   a. Z = lc

      1 = density

      c = ν of sound in that material.

      – As sound passes from one tissue plane to another, the amount of reflection is determined by the differences in the impedance of the two tissues.
      – Greater the difference, the greater the Z reflected.
      – Soft tissue—air—total reflection.
      – Soft tissue—bone—major amount is reflected.

   b. ∠ of insonation: The amount of reflection depends on the L between the sound beam and the reflecting surface.

      Best is, if its vertical the interface or within 3° from the ......

      There are 2 types of reflectors/echo producing mechanism.

      1. Specular—From smooth surfaces—Mirror like reflection

         —Produces strong directional echoes.

2. Scattering or Diffuse—Interference pattern from small parenchymal discontinuities. Each irregular points act as point couree. It produces weak, non-directional echoes.

2. Refraction:

- When sound waves pass from one medium to another, there is a change in the direction of the sound wave.
- It causes misregistration of a structure in the ultrasound image—leading to:

  – Spatial distortion.

  – Poor resolution.

3. Attenuation: Absorption is the loss of ultrasonic energy as heat while it passes through a medium.

Attenuation is total propagation loss.

Includes:

– Absorption.

– Scattering.

– Reflection.

Attenuation depends on:

– The insoating ν.

– Nature of the medium.

– Relaxation time.

High ν → more rapidly attenuated than low.

High density → more attenuation.

5

Computed Tomography

Basic Principles

The fundamental concept of CT is that the internal structure of an object can be reconstructed from multiple projections of the object. The final image is simply the sum of the back projections of all the different angular views of interest is the buildup of the image as more and more views are projected into the image matrix. An accurate reconstruction require that the views are evolved with an appropriate edge enhancing prior to back projection.

A computed tomography (CT) image is a display of the anatomy of a thin slice of the body developed from multiple X-ray absorption, measurements made around the body's periphery. Unlike conventional tomography, in which the image of a thin section is created by blurring out information from unwanted regions, the CT image is constructed mathematically using data arising only from the section of interest. Generating such an image is confined to cross-sections of the anatomy that are oriented perpendicular to the axial elimination of the body. Reconstruction of the final image can be accomplished in any plane, but conventionally it is performed in the transaxial plane.

In its most basic form, the fundamentals of CT are the same as these for radiography and tomography. Each approach directs a source of ionizing radiation through an object to recreate an image of the original object based on the X-ray absorption of the object. The basic equation used is same for each:

$$I = I_O e - \mu \text{ x}$$

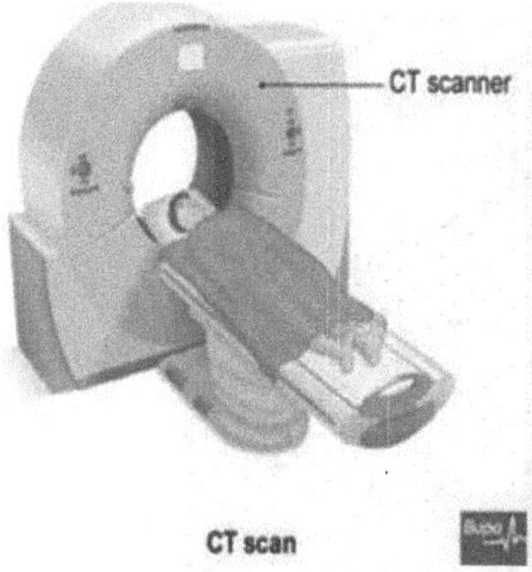

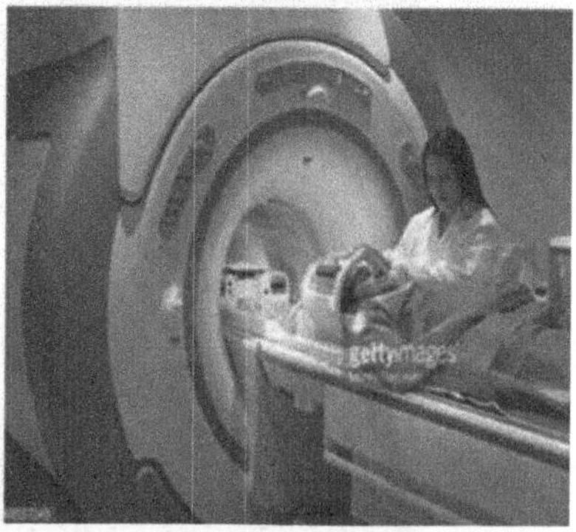

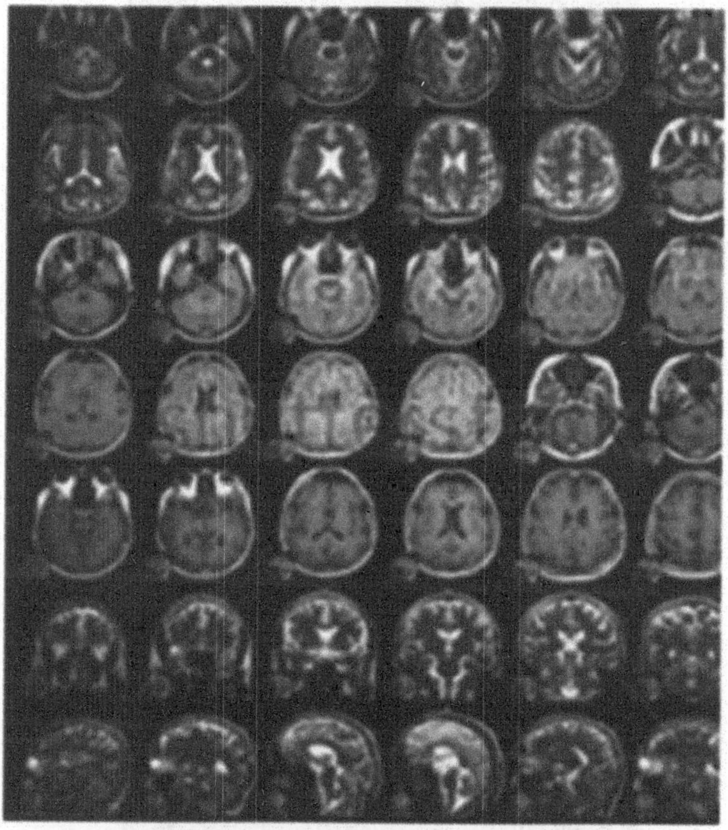

Fig. 5.1: Axial, coronal, sagittal section of brain of CT scan

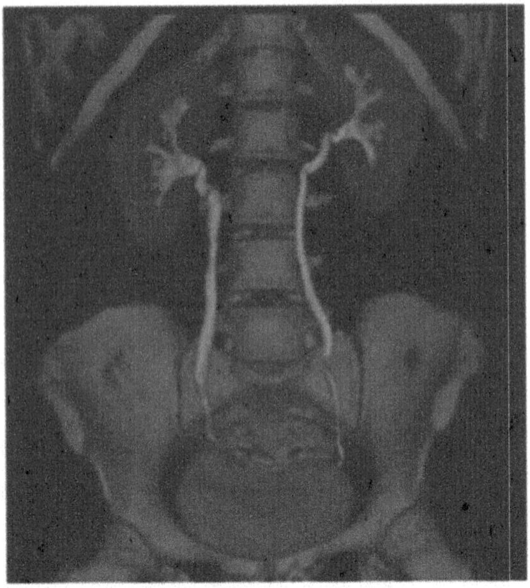

Fig. 5.2: CT–Urogram

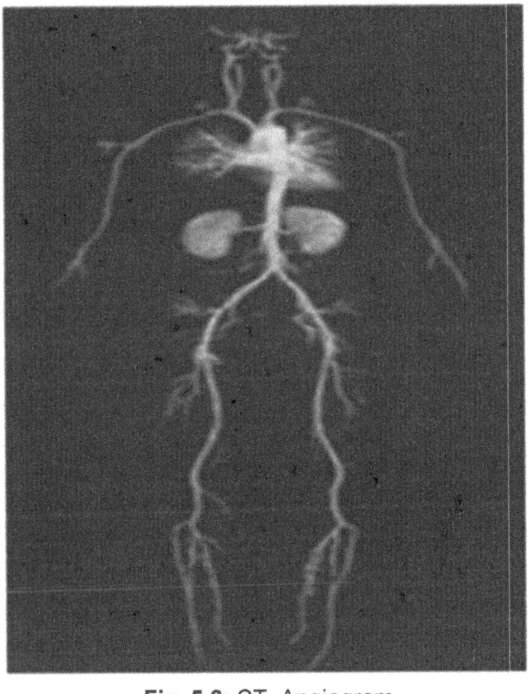

Fig. 5.3: CT–Angiogram

Where, I_0 : Is the incident intensity of an X-ray beam on the surface of an object of thickness, X.

I : Is the transmitted intensity.

e : Is Enler's constant (2.718).

μ : Is the linear attenuation coefficient.

The earliest CT was designed by Godfrey Hounsfield. The idea revolutionized the practice of radiology and helped Hounsfield to share of the Nobel prize.

The image reconstruction methodology described above is known as the filtered back-projection or convolution back projection algorithm. It was first applied to X-ray image reconstruction from projections in 1971 by Ramchandran and Lakshminarayanan. Subsequent improvements in the algorithm included the introduction of the Shepp and Logan Kernel, which minimized overshoot at abrupt patient attenuation differences, and the extensions to divergent X-ray projections. Of practical interest is that the first commercial CT scanner (EMI Mark I®) did not employ this algorithm initially but used an iterative algorithm. EMI Mark I head scanner was introduced in 1972.

The reconstructed image is a two-dimensional array of quantized gray scale values or pixels. There pixel values are directly related to the linear attenuation coefficients of the corresponding volume element of the slice:

Pixel value (Hounsfield Units, HU)

$= 1000\ (4\ \mu/\mu w - 1)$

Where, μ – is the average linear attenuation coefficient of the volume element represented by the pixels, and

μw – is a linear attenuation coefficient of water for the effective energy of the beam exiting the patient.

Thus water has a CT number of '0' and a region with a CT number of 100 HU has a linear attenuation coefficient that is 1% greater than the linear attenuation coefficient of water.

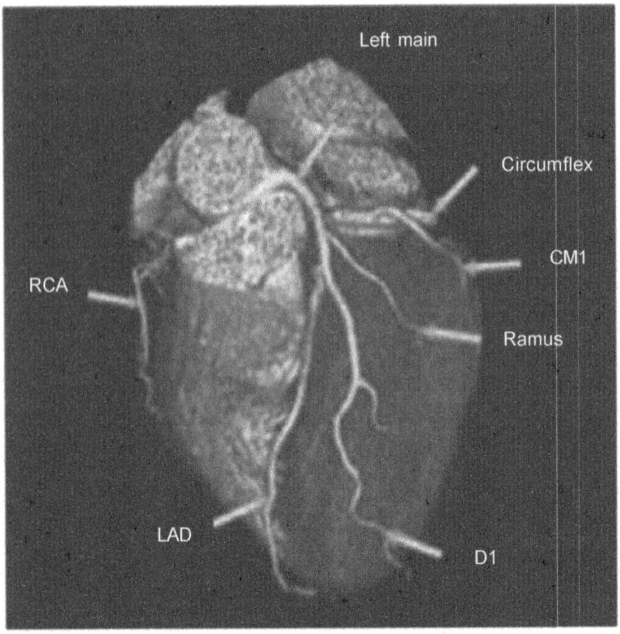

Fig. 5.4: CT–Coronary artery study

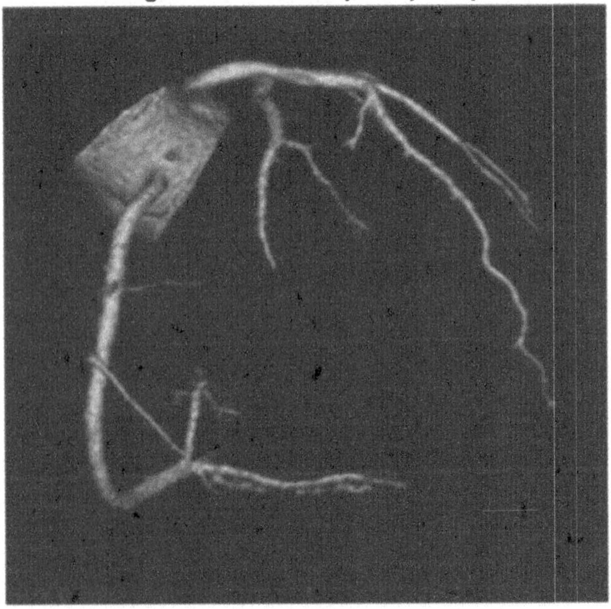

Fig. 5.5: CT–Coronary angiography. Software assisted coronary arteries

The pixel dimension is related to the display field of view (FOV) and the image matrix size.

$$\text{Pixel size} = \frac{\text{FOV}}{\text{Matrix size}}$$

CT images typically have a 12 bits per pixel, and these bits are used to represent numbers from – 1000 to 3095, a total of 2^{12} or 4096 different gray scale values. *Air* typically has a CT number of – 1000, Fat in the range of – 80 to – 100. *Soft tissue structures:* 10 to 80, and *bones:* 400 to 3000.

The number of a given type of the time will vary slightly from scanner manufacturer to manufacturer and will also be a function of the KV on a given scanner if the X-ray tube voltage is variable.

All the CT systems use a similar three step process to generate a CT image:

1. Scan, or data acquisition.
2. Reconstruction.
3. Display.

Evolution of Data Acquisition Systems and CT System Geometry

First Generation System

First generation CT data acquisitions was based on parallel beam geometry with a translate rotate principle of the tube/detector combination. The X-ray beam was collimated to dimensions of roughly 2 × 13 mm. The 13 mm dimension corresponded to the slice thickness (voxel length). Small detectors monitored the intensity of the beam before entering the body to yield the value of the incident intensity (I_0). After passing through the body, the beam was detected by a scintillation crystal, collimated to receive, primarily, those photons that were not scattered or absorbed. The amount of transmitted intensity (I) was then recorded and stored in the computer memory.

The X-ray tube and detector system were moved continuously across the patient, making 160 multiple measurements during the translation. At the end of each translation, the X-ray tube and detector system were rotated 1 degree and the translation repeated. The 160 measurements made during one complete translation are called a profile or view.

The first generation machine had the major disadvantage of long scanning times. Image quality severely suffered from the effects of patient motion, since 5 minutes were required to gather the 28,800 ray sums. This disadvantage limited the use for body parts such as the head, which can be made immobile.

Second Generation System

Second generation data acquisition and scanner geometry included fan beam reconstruction with a linear detector array. The X-ray beam was converted to fan shape with a diverging angle of between 3 and 10 degrees.

Multiple X-ray detectors were then placed adjacent to each other to intercept this beam. Now a scan can be obtained in period as short as 18 seconds. From the above figure, it is obvious that each detector obtains a different view during a translation because the rays from the X-ray tube to the detectors are not parallel.

Third Generation System

Third generation data acquisition and scanner geometry use wide-angle from beam geometry (50 to 55 degrees); an arc of detectors and an X-ray tube rotate continuously around the patient for 360°.

As the X-ray tube and detector arc are rotated, projection data (or data samples) are obtained and for every fixed point of the tube and detector, a view is created. The typical number of detectors ranges from about 600 to more than 900.

Fourth Generation System

Fourth generation data acquisition and scanner geometry also use a wide angle rotating fan beam (50 to 55°); in this case, through the

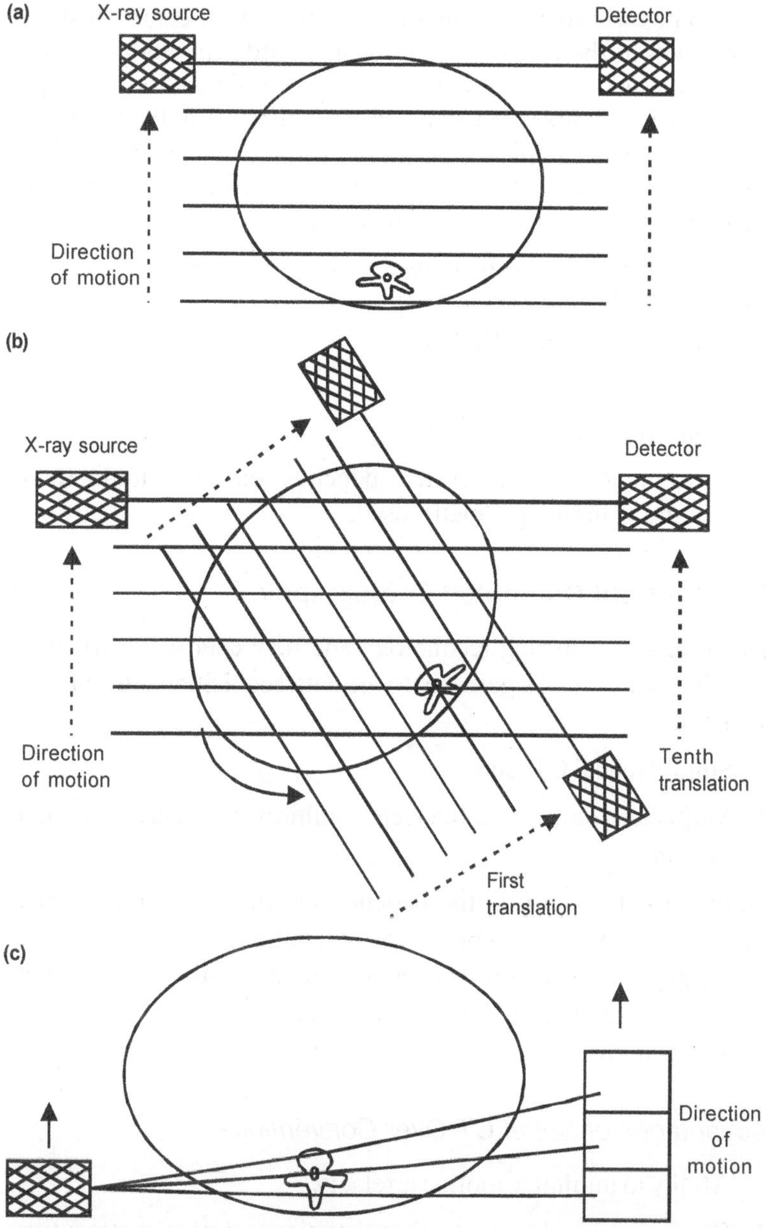

Figs 5.6a to c: Translate rotate scanner—(a) Original single detector system, single detector system or single translation; (b) Two separate

tube rotates within a 360° arc of the stationary detectors. Instead of the spots as the focus of views, as in a third generation system, views are seen from the perspective of the detectors with this approach data samples are obtained over the width of the fan angle and several data samples are acquired per detector. The output of each detector constitutes a view. Therefore, views are limited to the number of detectors in the 360° arc.

These are unique *advantages and disadvantages* in today's CT geometry beyond special resolution including:

1. Detected quantum efficiency.
2. Noise.
3. Contrast resolution.

Performance of each system depends, on the manufacturer and not the scanning geometry used.

Spiral/Helical Computed Tomography

The advent of slip ring technology and new data reconstruction techniques provided a gateway to the data acquisition currently in use namely:

1. Spiral/Helical CT; and
2. Multislice spiral or multidetector/multirow CT data acquisition systems.

In spiral/Helical CT, the patient table translates through the gantry while the X-ray tube (fourth generation) or the X-ray tube/ detector combination (third generation) rotate continuously around the patient, creating a volume of data. This permits new options in reconstruction.

Advantages of Spiral CT Over Conventional CT

1. Ability to minimize motion artefacts.
2. Decreased incidence of misregistration between consecutive axial slices.

3. Reduced patient dose.
4. Improved spatial resolution in the z-axis.
5. Enhanced multiplanar (MPR) or three dimensional (3D) rendering.

The ability to minimize motion artefacts in spiral CT is due to the faster scan times associated with every examination and the ability for many spiral CT examinations to be completed in a single patient breath-hold.

Multislice Spiral CT

The latest development in data acquisition-multislice spiral CT overcomes the limits of spiral CT. All multislice spiral CT systems today use third generation geometry (rotate only) with the added dimension of multiple arcs of detectors. The first deployment of this technology included a dual arc detector.

Four Slice Design

Since the introduction of dual detector technology in the early 1990s, other manufacturers have introduced four slice configurations. Two four slice design approaches are:

- Equal width detector.
- Variable width detector.

Display

Image display includes all of the system components necessary to connect the digital data provided by the reconstruction system to electrical signals used by the CT display monitor (cathode ray tube) or flat panel (liquid crystal display), enabling a graphic display of individual CT numbers representing attenuation values of individual sections of anatomy.

Further developments has resulted in 16 slice, 64 slice and 256 slice CT scan which basically helps in screening the cardiac pathology especially coronary artery disease and 3D vascular study. Also it helps in followup of coronary artery disease in its post therapy status. The various indications for 16 slice onward CT scan are following:

- **Gr I:** *Asymptomatic persons with the following risk factors:*
  - High BP (>130/90).
  - Diabetes.
  - High cholesterol (undiagnosed, >200 mg/dl).
  - Family history of heart disease.
  - Smoker.
  - Sedentary lifestyle (exercise less than three times a week).
  - Overweight by 20% or more.
  - High stress lifestyle.
  - Age: Men over 40 years old; women over 45 years old.
- **Gr II:** *Symptomatic persons:*
  - Detection and characterization of coronary artery occlusive lesion due to atherosclerosis, transplant arteriopathy and vasculitis.
  - Followup assessment of bypass grafts, stent patency.
  - Detection and characterization of coronary arteries anomalies, aneurysm etc.
  - Functional cardiac assessment.
  - Characterization of congenital heart disease.
  - Detection of cardiac masses, pericardial diseases.

Advantages and Disadvantages of CT

There are several advantages of using CT.

1. It completely defines the structures in the area of interest in the image with that of the other superimposition images.

2. Differences between the tissues with varying densities placed closely having a physical difference of less than 1% can be differentiated due to inherent property of high-contrast resolution.
3. The data collected from the volume of the tissue exposure can be presented and viewed in different planes of the body according to the requirement for the diagnostic purposes.
4. Improved resolution can be taken in comparison with the conventional radiography without using of the invasive procedures for example insertion of the catheter in angiography and in many cases of barium enema.
5. Reducing of the exposure dose to the patient as most of the modern systems are having very less exposure timing. It reduces the amount of exposure dose, as by taking a single scan and getting maximum information.
6. It can be used in medicine as a diagnostic tool and as a guide for interventional procedures with the help of contrast material. It is useful for highlighting structures, such as blood vessels. Use of contrast material can also helps in obtaining functional information about the tissues.

Apart from the above there are certain adverse effects of using CT:

1. Increases the radiation dose, if only a single conventional radiography solves the problem and the diagnosis can be done.
2. In certain patients the CT scan is contraindicated, to avoid the radiation dose and may lead to cancer. The most common cancers caused by CT are thought to be colon cancer, leukaemia and lung cancer in young people and women.

USE OR INDICATIONS OF CT SCANNING

Used to Detect:

1. Bleeding and brain substance injury as well as fracture of skull bones; in a case of head injury.

2. Bleeding caused by a ruptured or leaking aneurysm in a patient with a sudden severe headache.
3. Blood clot or bleeding within the brain shortly after a patient exhibits symptoms of a stroke.
4. Causes of stroke, especially with a new technique called perfusion CT.
5. Brain tumor.
6. Enlarged brain cavities (ventricles) in hydrocephalus.
7. Disease or malformation of the skull.
8. Evaluate the extent of bone and soft tissue damage in patients with facial trauma and help planning surgical reconstruction.
9. Diagnose disease of the temporal bone of skull which may be causing hearing problem.
10. Determine whether inflammation or other changes are present in the paranasal sinuses.
11. Plan radiation therapy for cancer of the brain.
12. C.T. helps to the passage of a needle used to obtain a tissue sample (biopsy) from the brain.
13. Useful to assess aneurysms or arteriovenous malformation through a technique called C.T. angiography.

HOW DO I PREPARE THE PATIENT

1. The patient should be explained about procedure.
2. Provide fitting clothing for patient at the time of examination.
3. Venflam fitting in antecubital vein to inject contrast media or treat the complication if any.
4. No contrast administration in cases with head injury.
5. Head injury will be entertained immediately and without any preparation.
6. For contrast study, patient needs at least 3 – 4 hours fasting.

7. Find out any history of heart disease, asthma, diabetes, kidney disease or thyroid disorder.
8. Whether the woman is pregnant. If yes, do not do the test because radiation effect to fetus.

HOW DOES THE EQUIPMENT LOOK LIKE?

C.T. scanner is large, box-like machine with a hole or short tunnel in the centre. Patient lie on a narrow examination table that slides into and out of this tunnel. X-ray tube rotates around the patient and electronic X-ray detectors are located opposite each other in a ring; called a gantry. The computer work station that processes the imaging information located in a separate control room, where the technician or radiologist operates the scanner and monitors the whole examination under direct visual contact and usually with the ability to hear and talk to the patient with the use of a speaker and microphone.

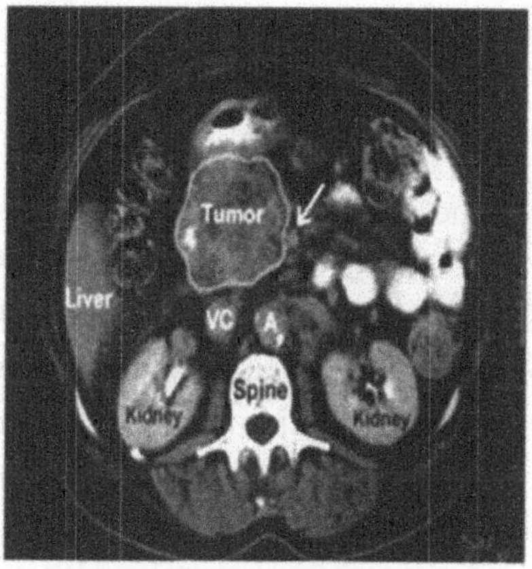

Fig. 5.7: CT abdomen

Here different body parts absorb X-ray in varying degrees. It is this crucial difference in absorption that allows the body parts to be distinguished from one another on an X-ray film or CT electronic image.

With CT scanning, numerous X-ray beams and a set of electronic X-ray detectors rotate around the patient measuring the amount of radiation being absorbed throughout the patient's body.

The examination table will move during the scan so that the X-ray beam follows a spiral path. A special computer program processes this large volume of data to create two dimensional cross sectional images of the body which then displayed on a monitor. CT imaging can be compared as to looking into a loaf of bread by cutting the loaf into thin slices. When the image slice are reassembled by computer software, the result is a very detailed multidimensional view of the body's interior.

Further advancement in detector technology allow all CT scanner to obtain multiple slices in a single rotation. These scanners are called as multi slice or multi-detector CT and allow thinner slices to be obtained in a shorter period of time. Modern CT scanners are so fast that they can scan through large section of body in just few seconds and even faster in small children, elderly and critically ill patient. For some CT examination contrast media may have to be used for enhancement the visibility.

Actual Procedure on Machine

The technician ask the patient to lie on the CT table on his/her back. Straps and pillows may be used to help maintain the correct position and to help the patient remain still during the examination.

Faster scanner help children to be scanned without sedation. However in special cases, sedation may be required for children who cannot hold still. Motion will cause blurring and degrade the contrast and brightness of the image.

After proper positioning, the table is allowed to more quickly through the scanner to determine the correct position for the scan. Then the table slowly move through machine when exposure is provided.

The patient is asked to hold the breath during scanning. Any motion whether breathing or body movements can lead to artifacts on the image.

After the examination is over, the patient is asked to wait till technician signals O.K. for desired contrast of image on computer.

Sometimes patient may experience pain, claustrophobia which may need some medication suggested by Radiologist.

Intravenous contrast is injected after plain CT scan to see enhancement of image in non-traumatic patient. Intravenous contrast injection may give rise to pin-prick sensation, feeling of warmth, flushed sensation, metallic test in mouth lasting for a minute or two. If patient feels the sensation to urinate and can't wait, then allow to urinate.

During exposure, nobody should be allowed in CT room. However, if circumstance arise then ask the attendant to cover himself by lead apron provided by department, this is needed especially when patient is small child.

If contrast media has been given, then after completion of examination remove the venflam and pressure is applied for some time, i.e., 5–10 minutes to stop the bleeding from injection site.

For chest examination, thin scan is obtained and is called as high resolution CT (HRCT) to delineate more detailed view of pulmonary alveoli and bronchopulmonary segmentation. To study pulmonary vasculature, pulmonary angiogram is obtained.

For abdominal CT scan, oral contrast media (Gastrografin or Trazogastro) mixed with 1.5 – 2 litre Bislary water is given to drink within 2 hours. of span. This visualizes the whole gastrointestinal tract. Simultaneously intravenous contrast media is injected through antecubital vein to study hepatic, renal splenic vasculature and even aorta and its branches. To study large bowel, contrast enema through rectal route also may be given, whenever necessary.

Advantage of CT Scan

1. It is painless, non-invasive and accurate procedure.
2. Able to image bony anatomy, soft tissue, blood vessel all at same time.

3. Provides detail image of many types of tissue as well as lung, bones and blood vessels.
4. The process is fast and simple in emergency cases. Reveal internal injuries and bleeding quickly to save life.
5. Cost – effective imaging technique.
6. Less sensitive to patient movement than MRI.
7. Unlike MRI. CT scan can be done even in patient with metallic implant.
8. CT avoids exploratory laparotomy and surgical biopsy.
9. No radiation remains in body after examination.
10. No side effect.

Risks:

1. Minimal chances of cancer due to high dose radiation.
2. Womon are advised to tell the radiologist whether she is pregnant.
3. Breast feed is prohibited to baby for 24 – 48 hours if contrast has been given.
4. Serious allergic reaction may occur with iodine containing contrast. Nowadays non-ionic contrast is used.

Limitation:

1. No absolute contraindication.
2. Very large head circumference in relation with Gantry window in conventional CT or over weight patient.
3. Compared to MRI, precise details of soft tissue (Brain) are less visible on CT scan. It is not sensitive in detecting inflammation of meninges.

6

PET–CT

Positron emission tomography–computed tomography (better known as PET–CT or PET/CT) is a nuclear medicine technique, combined in a single gantry, a positron emission tomography (PET) scanner and an X-ray computer tomography (CT) scanner, to acquire

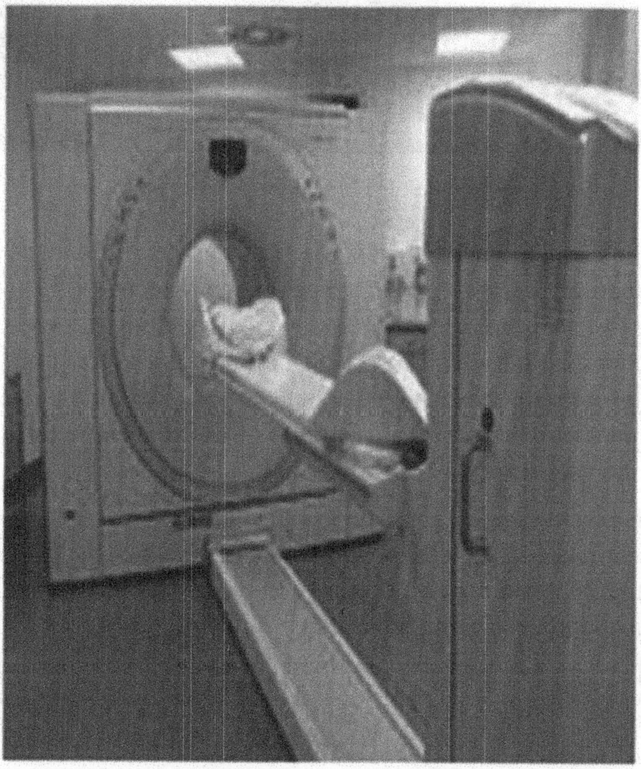

Fig. 6.1: PET – CT machine

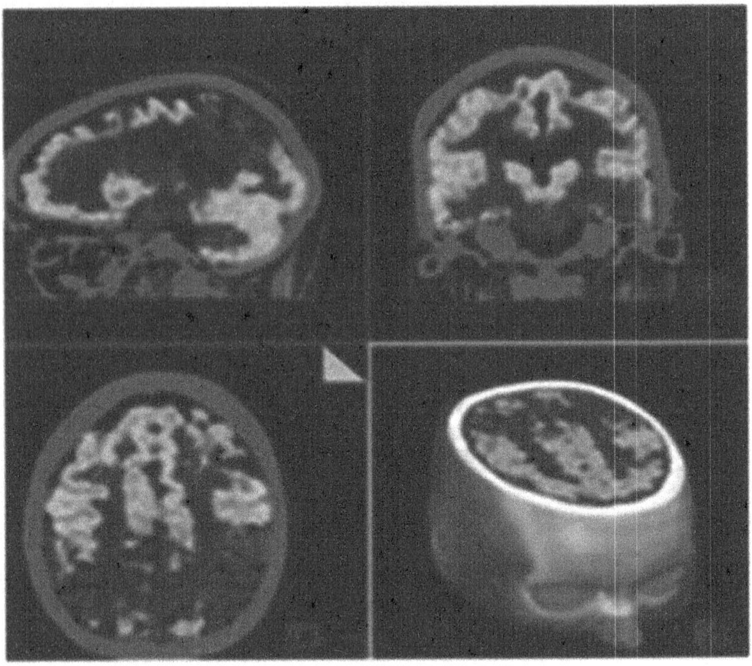

Fig. 6.2: PET/CT brain scan

sequential image from both devices in same session which are combined into a single superimposed image. Functional imaging obtained by PET, which depicts the spatial distribution of metabolic or biochemical activity in the body more precisely aligned or correlated with anatomic imaging obtained by CT scanning. 2–D or 3–D dimensional image reconstruction may be rendered as a function of common software and control system.

PET–CT has revolutionized medical diagnosis by adding precision of anatomic localization to functional imaging, which was lacking from pure PET imaging. These conventional PET scanner is either being abandoned or being replaced by PET–CT.

Only obstacle to wider use of PET–CT is difficulty and cost of producing and transporting the radiopharmaceuticals used for PET imaging which are extremely short lived (the half–life of radioactive fluorine–18) used to trace glucose metabolism using fluorodeoxy-glucose (FDG) is 2 hours only.

PET–MRI like PET–CT combines modalities to produce Co–registered image. PET–CT system was proposed by David Townsend (University of Geneva) and Ronald Nutt. First PET – CT prototype for clinical evaluation was installed at the university of Pittsburgh Medical Centre in 1998. The first commercial system reached the market in 2001.

Pre-requisites:

- At least 6 hours fasting is required.
- On the day of examination, the patient is asked to lie for minimum of 15 minutes in order to quite down the muscular activity which might be interpreted as abnormal metabolism.
- Low carbohydrate diet for previous 24 hours of date of examination.
- During pregnancy test is not done.
- Do not eat or drink anything except water as much as one can 6 hours prior to examination.
- Routine medicine if advised, may be taken.
- Anti–diabetic medicine be taken not less than 4 hours prior to examination.
- The patient is required to fill up the contrast screening form.

Procedure:

- An I.V. bolus injection of recently produced 2–FDG or 3–FDG is given through antecubital vein. The dose range from 3.7–7.4 megabecquerels (0.1 to 0.2 mci) per kg. body weight.
- The patient is brought to PET–CT device, lying in supine position with arm resting at the sides, or brought together above the head, depending on the main region of interest.
- The operation uses the PET–CT computer console to identify the patient and examination, delimit the caudal and rostral limit of body scan on to the scout view, select scanning parameters and starts image–acquisition period.

- The patient is automatically moved head first into the gantry and X-ray tomogram is acquired.
- Now the patient is automatically moved through PET gantry which is mounted in parallel with CT gantry and the PET slices are acquired.
- Patient now leave the device, and PET–CT software starts reconstructing and aligning the PET and CT image.
- During exposure patient needs to hold breath for short period.
- Patient may talk with technologist during examination.

A whole body scan from mid–thigh to top of head, takes 5–40 minutes depending upon acquisition protocol and technology of the equipment used. FDG imaging protocols acquire slices with a thickness of 2–3 mm. Hypermetabolic lesion are shown as false color coded pixels or voxels onto the gray value coded CT images. It provides qualification of size of lesion.

For uses in image guided radiation therapy of cancer, special fiducial marker are placed in the patient's body before acquiring PET–CT images. The slices thus acquired may be transferred digitally to a linear accelerator, needed to perform precise bombardment of the target areas using high energy photons (radiosurgery).

PET in cancer allows to see the cancer metabolizes, spread or metastasis to new areas and tumor response to chemotherapy.

Contraindication:

1. Not done in pregnant woman and breastfeeding female.
2. May be harmful in patient of kidney disease or with raised creatinine level from medicine being taken.

Adverse Reaction:

1. Claustrophobia.
2. Uncomfortable with needles.

3. Allergic reaction.
4. Buzzing and clicking noise during reaction.

After the Procedure:

- Should drink 5 glass of water.
- Nursing mother should start breastfeeding only after 24 hours.
- May feel nasal congestion, nausea, vomiting, dizziness itchy eye, hives, rashes, sneezing, restlessness, tremor, pain etc. Inform the staff, who will take care of the problem.
- Tracer will be out after 2 days.

7

Magnetic Resonance Imaging

Magnetic resonance (MR) is a phenomenon involving magnetic fields and radiofrequency (RF) electromagnetic waves. It was discovered in 1946 independently by Bloch and co-workers at Stanford and by Purcell at Harvard. Since then magnetic resonance imaging (MRI) has been a useful tool, especially for analytical chemistry and biochemistry. MRI uses electromagnetic radiation to probe inside the human body but radiation has low energy and appears safe under normal operating conditions. Jackson (1967) first utilised MR signals for human study. Gabillard investigated one-dimensional (1D) distribution of MR signal. Lauterber (1972) could generate 2-D proton MR image for the first time. In 1974 Lauterbur produced the first image of a live animal.

T_1 Relaxation

RF stimulation causes nuclei to absorb energy, lifting them to the excited state. The nuclei return to the ground state by dissipating their excess energy to their surrounding, which is called the lattice. This process "spin lattice relaxation" describes the recovery of the longitudinal magnetization toward its equilibrium value. It depends on the lattice having a magnetic field that fluctuates at the Larmor frequency. Such a fluctuating magnetic field comes from rotation and translation of the nuclei in molecules of the lattice undergoing Brownian Motion. Average frequency of this motion depends upon the size of molecules in the lattice. The frequency of rotation in medium size molecules such as lipids is closest to typical Larmor

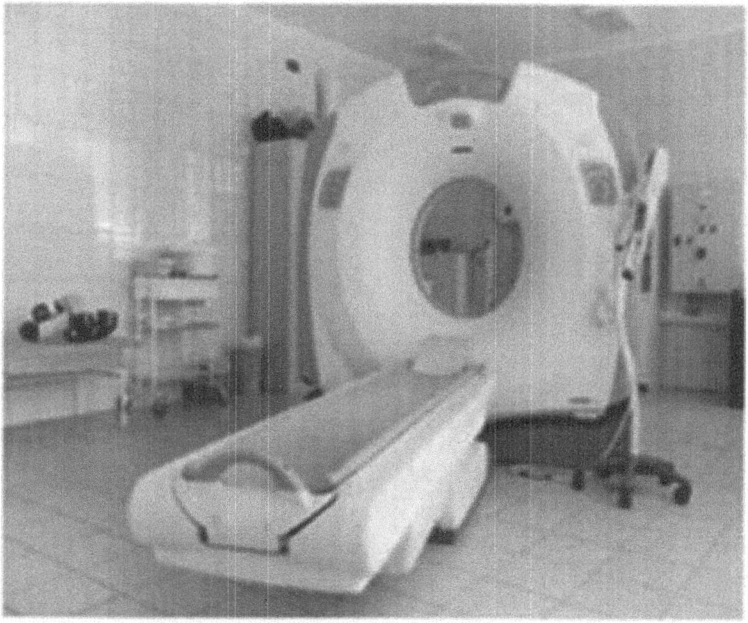

Fig. 7.1: MRI machine

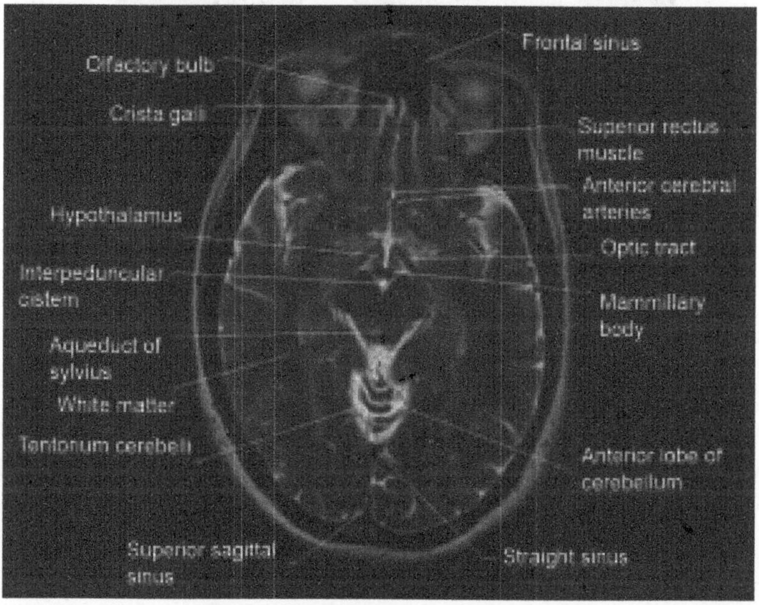

Fig. 7.2: Axial study of brain on MRI

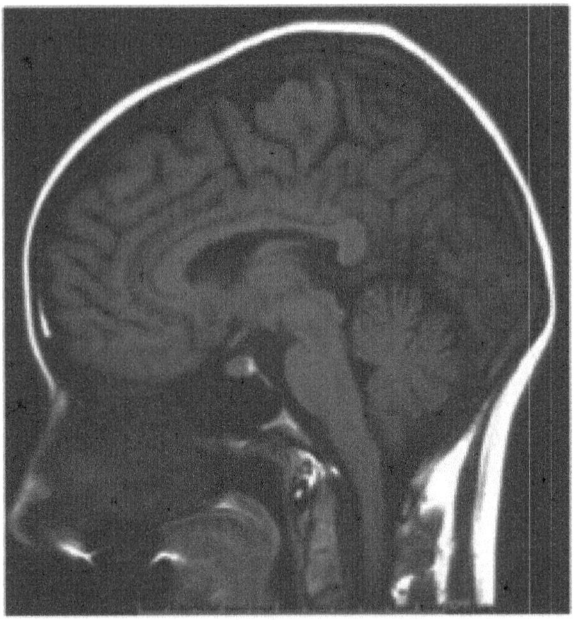

Fig. 7.3: Sagittal section of brain on MRI

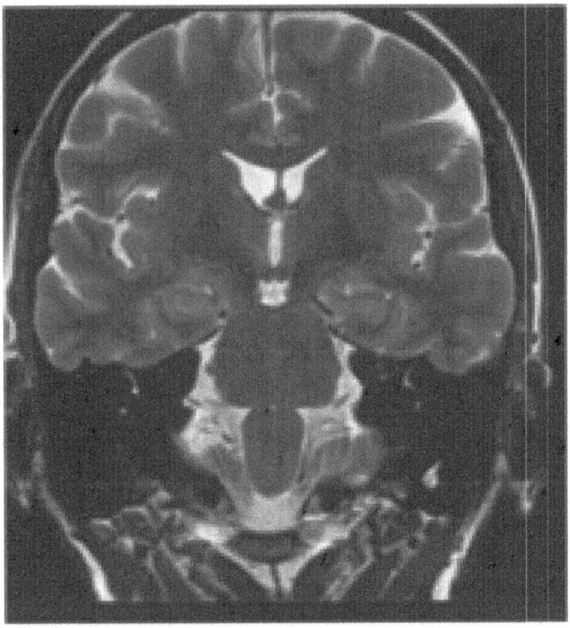

Fig. 7.4: Coronal view brain on MRI

frequency. Therefore magnetization associated with lipids relaxes faster than that associated with pure water or much larger molecules such as protein. T_1 relaxation times depend on magnetic field strength because the latter affects the Larmor frequency.

T_2 Relaxation

Transverse magnetization decays because its component magnetic movements get out of phase as a result of their mutual interaction. Anything that changes the magnetic field strength also changes the precessional frequency and causes a loss of phase coherence and shrinkage of transverse magnetization. A process called T_2 relaxation denotes the "loss of phase coherence" caused by interaction between neighbouring magnetic moments.

Unlike T_1 relaxation, no energy is transferred from nuclei to the lattice in T_2 relaxation. Large molecules which tend to reorient more slowly than small molecule, promoter T_2 relaxation and have shorter T_2 time. Free water has a longer T_2 than water associated with macromolecules, the magnetic field strength influence T_2 much less than T_1.

Repetition Time: The time between repeated RF excitation pulses is called the repetition time (TR).

Slice Selection

Mechanism: Slice selection combines a magnetic field gradient and a specially shaped RF pulse to restrict MR signal to a slice instead of entire region influenced by the transmitter coil, the gradient spreads out the Larmor frequency so that frequencies contained in the RF pulse affect only a slice.

Slice Orientation: Orientation of a slice depends on 3 magnetic field gradient is activated during RF pulse. If a patient is positioned head first and supine in a magnet, RF pulse in presence of Z gradient creates a transverse slice, the 'X' and 'Y' gradients select slice in sagittal and coronal orientation respectively. Oblique slices are created by activating two or more gradients during on RF pulse.

Slice Position: Slice are rotated where the Larmor frequency matches the frequency of RF pulse. Slice selection gradient lowers the Larmor frequency on one side of centre of magnet and raises it on other side. Slice position is controlled by changing the frequency of RF pulse because changing the amplitude of slice selection gradient would inadvertently alter the thickness of slice.

Slice Thickness and Profile

RF pulses perturb magnetization within a band of Larmor frequencies matching the frequencies contained within RF pulse which is called its bandwidth; which depends on shape and duration of RF pulse. Longer RF pulses which have a lower band width produce thinner slices.

Instruments

- The key components of an MR system are the magnet, the gradient, the radiofrequency subsystem and the computer.
- The magnet can be superconducting, resistive or permanent. Superconducting magnets tend to have high fields in Tesla and therefore higher signal to noise. Resistive and permanent magnets tend to have a more open architecture, allowing interventional MRI applications and reduced claustrophobia.
- The gradients are resistive electromagnets consisting of metallic coils driven by power amplifiers. Gradient performance is measured in amplitude and rise time, larger values of the former and small values of the latter being required for high performance applications.
- The RF system consists of a transmitter, a receiver, and coils which can be simple surface coils, double saddle cools quadrature-receive/quadrature excitation coils or phased array coils.

The computer is required for data manipulation and to co-ordinate the RF and gradient system (Flowchart 7.1).

- Most of the contrast in MR images comes from variations in relaxations time T_1 and T_2.
- T_1 is the longitudinal or spin lattice, relaxation time. It is longer in pure water than in proteinaceous solution or tissues or when paramagnetic species capable of dipole-dipole interactions are present. T_1 is a first order exponential time constant that reflects the molecular tumbling rate of protons and the strength of local magnetic fields they experience.
- T_2 is the transverse or spin-spin, relaxation time. It is also longer in pure water than in proteinaceous solution or tissues or when paramagnetic species capable of dipole-dipole interaction are present. T_2 is also shorter when protons exchange between different susceptibility. T_2 is also first order exponential time constant so that 63% of the initial transverse magnetization or signal is lost during one T_2 period.
- All MRI pulse sequence include a combination of H_2 spin density T_1 and T_2 contrast. The particular weighting of these inherent sources of tissue contrast is determined by RF pulse intensity "tip angles", pulse sequences and interpulse timing parameters.
- SE image T_1 weighting is determined by TR and T_2 weighting by TE, hydrogen spin density weightening is always present.
- Inversion recovery image T_1-weighting is determined by T_1 while TR has a minor effect and TE controls T_2 weighted contrast.
- Gradient echo image contrast is determined primarily by the tip angle Q. Short TR values permit rapid planar (2D FT) imaging and volume (3D FT) imaging.
- Statistical noise is usually more apparent at low magnetic field strengths. It can be minimized by increasing the number of acquisition per phase-encoding strep, by decreasing the band width, and by decreasing the sensitive volume of the receiver coil.

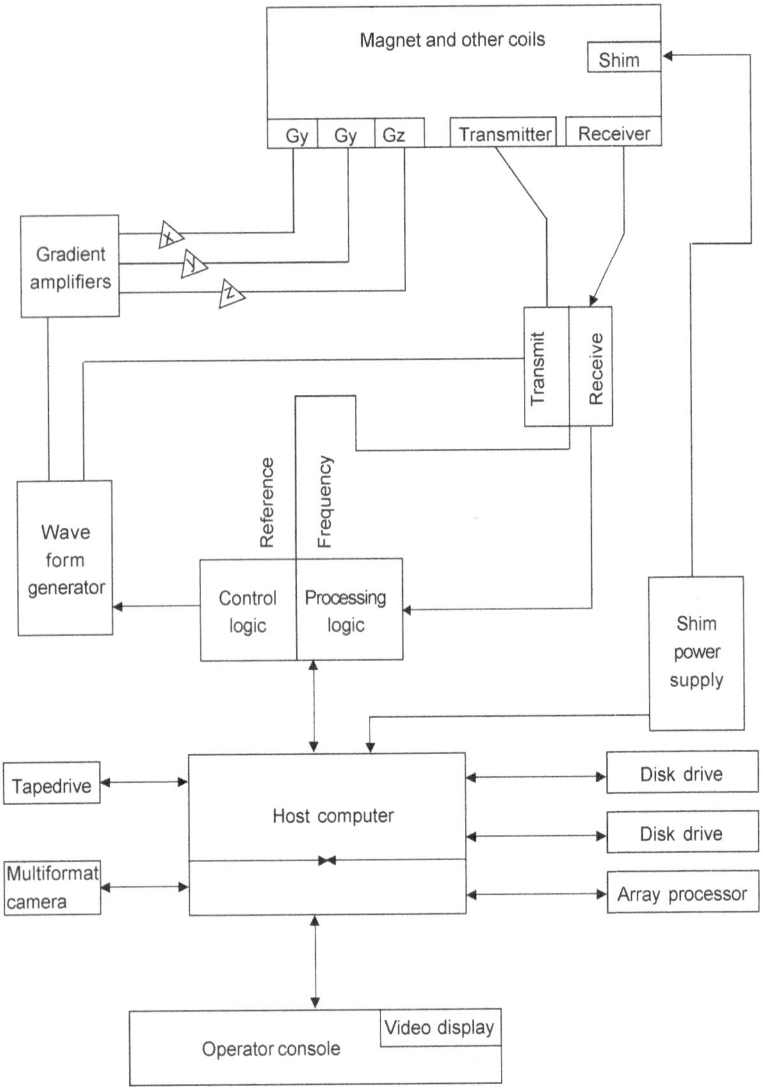

Flowchart 7.1: Simplified diagram of MR system

- Systematic noise is usually more apparent at high magnetic field strengths. It can be decreased by minimizing patient motion, by eliminating signal producing tissues lying outside the field of view in the acquired plane and by increasing the number of averages per phase-encoding step.
- Detection of pathology is improved by maximizing signal and contrast relative to noise.

  MR imaging is the multislice imaging, i.e., simultaneous excitation of adjacent slices while data from one slice is being acquired.

Classification of Pulse Sequences

1. *Spin-echo:*
   - Single echo
     - CSE (Conventional spin echo).
   - Multiecho
     - FSE (Fast spin echo).
     - TSE (Turbo spin echo).
     - RARE (Rapid acquisition relaxation enhancement).
2. *Gradient echo:*
   - Single echo
     - GRE (Gradient recalled echo)
       - # Spoiled.
       - # Refocussed.
   - Multi echo
     - EPI (Echo plannar imaging).

Characteristics of FSE: The signal characteristics of FSE are slightly different from CSE.

- The fat appears bright on T_2W images of FSE than the T_2W images of CSE.

- FSE is less sensitive to magnetic susceptibility effects. This is of advantage in imaging areas where artefacts due to presence of metallic foreign bodies are to be avoided. On the other hand, this is a disadvantage when imaging intracranial haemorrhage.
- The signal intensity of the FSE is more than expected, there is better contrast between the gray and white matter.

Clinical Application of FSE: FSE has replaced the CSE for T_2W images in most applications due to reduction in the scanning time and higher resolution. It has been used for brain, spine and musculoskeletal imaging and imaging of pelvis.

Inversion Recovery Pulse Sequences: Depending on the inversion time (TI) the sequence can be STIR (short time inversion recovery) or FLAIR (fluid attenuation IR). In STIR, the T_I is about 100 ms and in FLAIR, the T_I is very long about 2000 ms.

FLAIR is a significant advancement and is a powerful tool for demonstrating subtle lesions abutting CSF spaces, e.g., periventricular demyelinating plaques. It has become part of routine brain MR protocols.

The STIR images are used for fat suppression. They are used for the demonstration of optic nerve lesions and bone marrow pathology.

Gradient Echo Imaging: It uses low flip angle and short TR.

Uses of GRE

- It can be acquired in very short time with improved SNR per unit time. This sequence can be used to obtain T_1 (large flip angle and short TE), T_2 (small flip angle and large TE and short TE). TR is not very important for image contrast.
- The GRE images depend on the T_2. This is of advantage in imaging haemorrhage and calcifications. On the other hand, magnetic susceptibility artefact arising from a metallic foreign body and base of the skull can be problematic.

- This sequence is used for breathhold imaging of the abdomen, 3D imaging and for dynamic contrast enhancement.
- Rapid application of RF pulses in GRE causes saturation of the stationary material whereas the inflowing unsaturated blood appears hyperintense. This is the underlying principle of time of flight (TOF) angiography.

Variants of GRE

- SPGR—(Spoiled gradient echo).
- FLASH—(Fast low angle shot).
- FISP—(Fast imaging with steady procession).
- GRASS—(Gradient recalled acquisition into steady state).
- CISS—(Constructive interference in steady state).

Echoplanar Imaging (EPI)

It is the ultrafast imaging. This allows study of dynamic process and motion free images.

Magnetisation Transfer Contrast (MTC)

- It enhances the visibility of enhancing lesions and other short T_1 pathology.
- Quantitative studies, i.e., measurement of MTR (magnetisation transfer ratio) has a potential in assessment of severity score of multiple sclerosis and grading of tumors.

	T_1W–Short TR, Short TE	*T_2W–Long TR, Long TE*
Fluid	Black	Bright
Fat	Very bright	Intermediate
Muscles	Intermediate	Hypointense
Ligaments and tendon	Black	Black
Flowing blood	Signal void (black)	Signal void (black)
Gray matter	Gray	Hyperintense
White matter	White	Hypointense

Proton Density (PD)*—Long TR, Short TE*

Fluid	:	Intermediate
Ligament and tendon	:	Hypointense
Flowing blood	:	Signal void (Black)
White matter	:	Hypointense
Gray matter	:	Hyperintense

FLAIR:

Fluid	:	Black
Flowing blood	:	Signal void
White matter	:	Hypointense
Gray matter	:	Hyperintense
Fat	:	Intermediate

STIR:

Fat	:	Black
Flowing blood	:	Black

GRE:

Flowing blood	:	White

MTC:

Just like T_1W, but slow flowing blood (e.g. in sinuses) can appear bright.

MR Contrast Media

Use of intravenous contrast Gadolinium—DTPA began in 1983.

Criteria for Contrast Media

- They should alter the parameters responsible for image contrast in MRI.

- They should possess some tissue specificity.
- They should be substantially cleared from the targeted tissue in a reasonable period of time.
- They should have low toxicity and be stable in vitro.
- They must possess a suitable shelf life for storage.

Mechanism of Action

- Relaxivity—that affect:
  - T_1 relaxation: +ve relaxation agent.
  - T_2 relaxation: –ve relaxation agent (decreased T_2 means decreased signal on T_2WI).
- Susceptibility

  Four types of substances:
  - Ferromagnetic
  - Superparamagnetic.

  Paramagnetic substances afford greatest flexibility in contrast agent design and they can strongly influence the relaxation properties of nearby protons leading to changes in tissue contrast.
  - +ve T_1 relaxation contrast agent.
  - May affect T_2 at high concentration.

  Superparamagnetic substances produce magnetic field so their presence causes dephasing of protons of tissues leading to decrease T_2 time, i.e., signal loss (–ve signal on T_2WI).
- Diffusion and perfusion.

Gadolinium

Most common paramagnetic ion is gadolinium ion which is complexed with various chelates like DTPA, HP-D03A.

GD-DTPA—Presence of unpaired in the paramagnetic ion is important to affect change in relaxation of T_1/T_2. The magnetic dipole moment (MDM) created by the unpaired can enhance the relaxation rates of H_2O protons either by direct interaction with H_2O protons or by local magnetic field influence. This is relaxivity theory, i.e., leading to decreased T_1 time which causes increased signal on T_1WI. This could be either inner sphere relaxation or outer sphere relaxation.

Ligands/Chelates

Also affects the contrast agent design, like DTPA being a large molecule, the complex rotates more slowly and translates more slowly in space so increased interaction of Gd with H_2O protons hence decreased relaxation time.

It also causes increased distance between ion and H_2O proton which decreased relaxation affect.

But their use is important as gadolinium ions, alone when free in body cause high toxicity. These ligands cause rapid and total renal excretion and reduces toxicity.

Pharmacokinetics

After I.V. injection, Gadolinium circulates in the vascular system to be distributed in blood pool and extracellular spaces but does not cross the blood brain barrier (BBB) and excreted unchanged through kidney.

$$t½ = \sim 90 \text{ minute}$$

They cross the abdomen BBB thus being useful in detection of pathologies. They are useful in imaging of pathological processes in the enhancement dependent on vascular permeability.

MR-Relevant Paramagnetic Metals

- Fe^{3+}
- Mn^{2+}
- Gd^{3+}
- Dy^{3+}

Gd-chelates in use in USA approved by FDA

- HP-D03A
- DTPA-diethylene triamine petacetic acid.
- DTPA-BMA.

Approved in USA

Gd-DTPA: Gadopentate dimeglumine (Magnevist)—1st extracellular Gd chelate to be developed for clinical use.

Non-Ionic: Gd-HP D03A-Gadoteridol/Prohance.

Gd-DTPA-BMA: Gadodiamide/omniscan.

Other Gd Chelates:

Ionic: Gd-DOTA—Gadoterate meglumine.

Non-Ionic: Gd-D03A—Gadobutral Gadoversetamide.

Gd-BOMA: Gadobenate dimeglumine (Multihance).

Indications

More used in CNS and spine:
- Tumors.
- Infections.
- Activity in MS.
- Early detection of small neuromas and meningiomas.
- Leptomeningeal deposits.

Image Sequence:
- Conventional sequences.
- FSE.
- GRE.
- Perfusion/diffusion.

Type of MR Contrast Agents

1. Based on relaxation effects:

   +ve relaxation agents— Gd chelates
   Dys/chelates
   Mn agents

   –ve relaxation agents
2. Based on route of administration:

   I.V.

Oral —	+ve :	Gd DTPA
		Oil emulsion
	–ve :	Based of Fe particles
		Blue berry juice

3. Based on their location in the body:
   a. Extracellular.
   b. Blood pool agents.
   c. Liver contrast agent.
   d. Endoluminal.
4. Based on their physical properties:
   a. Non-particulate.
   b. Particulate
      - SIO (large SIO's).
      - Magnetite (small SIO).
      - Iron oxide Nanocolloids (Ultrasmall SIO's).

Gd-DTPA

- Is ionic charged.
- Approved for use in US by FDA in 1988.
- First extracellular Gd chelate in use.
- Adult and paediatric patient—0.1 mmol/kg (>2 years).
- Caution—In renal impaired patient.
  Removed by dialysis.
- Gd ion per se can cause hemolysis but with chelates not seen. Sometimes small amount of Gd^{+} ion may be released from chelates.
- Mild increase in serum Fl and bilirubin within 3 hours reaches peak between 6 and12 hours and returns to baseline after 24 hours.
- Safety in pregnancy—not known. It can cross placenta and secreted in breast milk.
- 3-5% rate of adverse reactions after I.V. administration.

- Majority:
  - Mild-nausea and
  - Anaphylactoid reactions very rare.
- Non-ionic
  - Lower osmolality.
  - Lower viscosity.
  - Higher stability of chelate in vivo.

Newer Applications

High Dose: 0.3 mmol/kg contrast study reveals improved enhancement, detection and delineation.

Magnetization transfer—Addition to MT pulses to standard imaging sequences can improve the visualisation of contrast enhancement in brain especially in infarction.

First pars studies—can be done on:

- Conventional 1.5 Tesla unit; or
- Newer echoplanar units.

Rapid dynamic imaging of the bolus of the contrast agent as it passes through the brain, one can assess γCBV and thus brain perfusion.

Higher dose study more useful.

MR Angiography

Flow-related enhancement is an enhancement of flowing blood seen on gradient echo pulse sequences as well as in entry slices of multislice spin echo sequences. This enhancement is a result of inflow of unsaturated (completely relaxed) spins into a slice plane or imaging volume between RF excitations. Stationary spins within the imaging volume will undergo incomplete T_1 relaxation between RF excitations resulting in less signal of following the next RF pulse when compared to inflowing, completely relaxed spins in flow blood. The distance that the unsaturated blood can extend into an imaging volume and therefore the degree of enhancement is proportional to

TR and the velocity of the blood. The use of gradient motion nulling (flow compensation) improves the flow-related enhancement in gradient echo sequences.

TOF MR Angiography (Time of Flight MR Angio)

With 3-D TOF, a volume of images are obtained simultaneously by phase-encoding in the slice-select direction. An angiographic appearance can be generated using MIP, as is done with 2-D TOF. Several 3-D TOF angiography will allow greater spatial resolution in the slice-select direction than 2-D TOF, however with thick volume and slow flowing blood, loss of signal is seen with 3-D TOF method.

Phase-Contrast MR Angiography

Spins that are moving in the same direction as a magnetic fluid gradient develop a phase shift that is proportional to the velocity of spins. This is the basis of phase-contrast angiography. Bipolar phase gradient used to encode the velocity of spins. Stationary spins undergo no net change in phase after the two gradients are applied. Moving spins will experience a different magnitude of the second gradient compared to the first, because of its different spatial position. This results in a net phase shift. This information can be used directly to determine the velocity of the spins. Alternatively, the image can be subtracted from one acquired without the velocity encoding gradients to obtain an angiogram.

Contrast enhanced angiography—Gadolinium chelates are used.

Functional MRI

Several 3-D TOF volumes can be combined to visualise longer segment of vessels. Functional MRI (FMRI) is a technique that has recently been introduced to obtain functional information from the central nervous system. FMRI may be useful for preoperative neurosurgical planning, epilepsy evaluation and brain trapping.

Newer Agents

More specificity needed so that they can remain in circulation for a longer time.

A. **Blood pool agents:** 3rd major class of MR contrast media. They reversibly bind to plasma albumin. Increased magnitude and duration in the circulation—increased plasma t½-allows more prolonged investigation time.

   Coated SPIO's, Gd complex with added coating.

   Specific use—For small vessels (coronary and accessory renal arteries).

   Vessels with slow flow—Deep vein thrombosis, pulmonary embolism.

   Vessels with complex flow pattern—AV malformation.

   Very much helps when imaging the moving targets like heart.

B. **Hepatobiliary Contrast Agents:**

   - Hepatocyte
     - Gd based: Gd BOPTA
       Gd-EOB BOPTA
     - Mn base: Mn DPDP.

Particulate Agents

- Iron particles of various size.
- Reaction rates are higher than Gd-Chelate.
- They are of various sizes and taken up by reticuloendothelial system (RES).
  - AMI-25
  - Magnetite
  - Ultrasmall-AMI 227

  They improve lesion detection rate.

Targeted Contrast Agents

Tissue or tumor specific contrast agents (i.e. blood pool agents, liver specific agents).

Latest developments are:
- Necrosis specific agents (Bis-Gd-mesoporphyrin).
- Lymphographic contrast agent.
- Agents targeted at inflammation detection.
- Liposomes as carriers.

Endoluminal Contrast Agents

Positive Contrast Agents:
- Paramagnetic agents—Gd-DTPA with or without mannitol ferric ammonium citrate (Geritol).
- Short T_1-relaxation agents—Mineral oil, oil emulsion—useful for stomach and small intestine only as absorbed in small bowel.
- Combination of above.

Negative Contrast Agents
- Diamagnetic agents—Kaolin, Barium sulphate.
- SPIO's—Magnetite albumin spheres, oral magnetic particles.
- Perfluorochemicals—It replaces protons by fluonne thus leading to absence of signal in bowel.
- PFOB—Rapid transit, lack of taste and odour so palatable, absence of any known side effect.

Advantages of Using of MRI
1. It does not make use of the radiations, hence minimizing the radiation dose to the patients.
2. It provides maximum contrast between soft tissues located close to each other with varying densities. It is useful in imaging brain, heart and muscles and can even diagnose cancers and its extent.
3. Three dimensional image can be formed and can be rotated at any dimension, i.e., can be viewed from all angles of the body.

Disadvantages
1. It cannot be used with the patients of metallic implants, including cochlear implants and cardiac pacemakers. These implants are attracted with the high magnetic fields.
2. It is contraindicated for the patients undergone open heart surgeries or any other surgeries in which metallic clips were used.

8

Mammography

Accurate assessment of the breast as to whether it is normal or not is foremost important.

The efficacy of diagnostic mammography depends upon:

- The optimal radiographic demonstration of breast.
- The perception of abnormal features.
- The correct interpretation of these findings. The diagnostic algorithm is as follows—are the appearances:
  - Normal.
  - Abnormal.

If abnormal, are they:

1. Benign:
   a. Benign breast change, tumors, cysts.
   b. Infections, haemorrhage or scars.
2. *Malignant:*
   Single, multifocal, multicentric, calcification.
3. *Equivocal:*
   Masses, stromal patterns, calcification.

Sensitivity of test defines the accuracy of the positive diagnosis in the positive detection rate.

Specificity of test indicates the rate of mammographic false positive diagnosis in women free of cancer in the screened population.

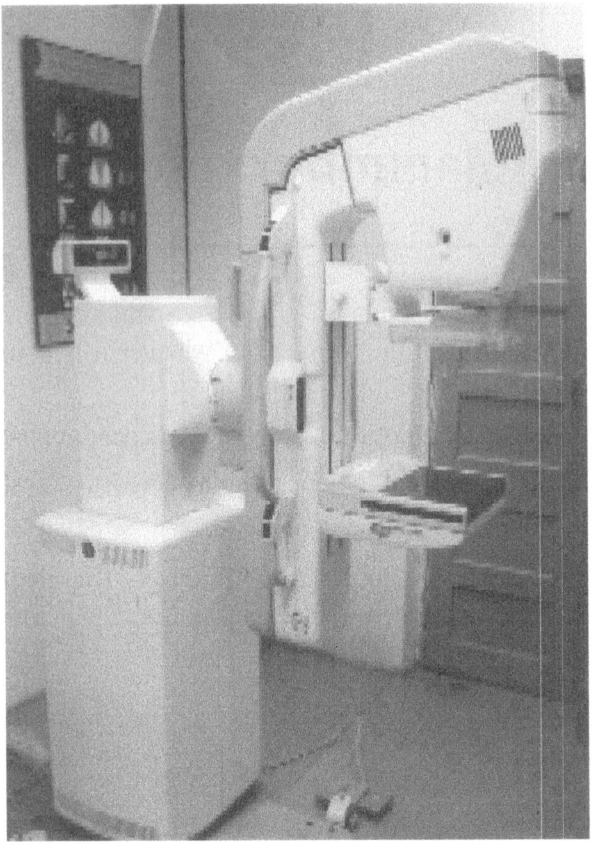

Fig. 8.1: Photograph of dedicated mammographic machine (DMR 80)

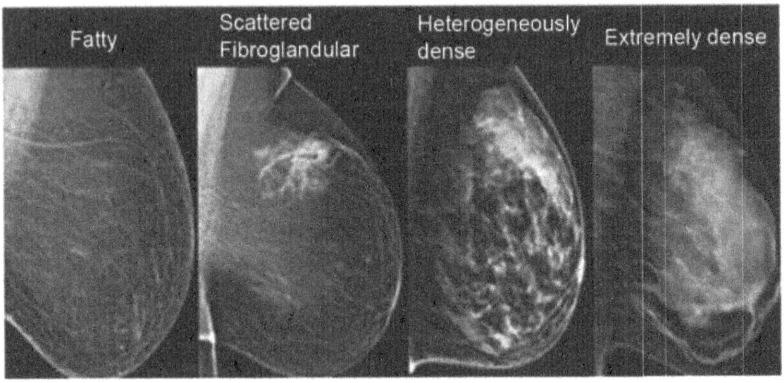

Fig. 8.2: Mammograph showing different type of breast pathologies

Sensitivity and specificity are inversely related. Higher sensitivity means that fewer cancers are missed. Higher specificity means that fewer false positive diagnosis are made.

In mammography there are four physical parameters that must be considered when assessing the performance of the imaging system:

1. Contrast—to see small differences in soft tissue density.
2. Resolution—to demonstrate as small as 100 μm microcalcification.
3. Dose.
4. Noise.

Components of the mammographic imaging system—mammographic X-ray set is a dedicated unit with a low energy X-ray spectrum and a small focal spot.

1. Compression device—Film compression is important in mammography because it reduces breast doses and prevents or reduces movements unsharpness but it also produces several other benefits. Geometric unsharpness is reduced. Image contrast is also improved.
2. Anti scatter grid.
3. Screen-film combination.
4. Digital receptors.
5. Automatic exposure control.

Mammography has been proved to be the single most important breast imaging technique both for symptomatic and asymptomatic women. In asymptomatic women, the purpose is to detect non-palpable abnormalities. Symptomatic women with a known palpable lump or a suspicious area of the breast require diagnostic problem-solving mammography.

It is important for the radiographer to mask on a diagram the site of skin lesions and scars. Identification letter should be placed in axillary region well away from the breast. Medial and axillary positional markers can also be placed on the film.

Even with good technique 5-10% of breast cancers are not detected by mammography. Inferior quality and poor positioning technique will limit the interpretation skills of the radiologist.

POSITIONING TECHNIQUE

When the compression plate is applied, some of the posterior portion of the breast is omitted from each view. The hemispherical shaped breast curves around the chest wall extending from lateral margin of the sternum to the axilla, and overlies the pectoral muscles. Although the mediolateral oblique view should demonstrate the maximum amount of glandular tissue, the geometry between the breast, the shape of the thoracic wall and the straight edge of the film support may make it difficult to project all the breast tissue in one view. It may therefore be necessary to take two or more views. Any lesion seen must be demonstrated in at least two views. Magnification or localized spot compression of the usual mammographic views may be required to evaluate specific areas within the breast.

Following are the views:

- Mediolateral oblique (MLO).
- Craniocaudal.
- Craniocaudal with lateral rotation.
- Craniocaudal extended.
- Craniocaudal semi extended.
- Craniocaudal medial quadrant.
- 30° oblique.
- Axillary.
- Lateral—mediolateral.
- Lateral—lateromedial.
- Specialized.
- Spot compression.
- Magnification.

Evaluation Criteria

See Figures 8.3a and 8.3b.

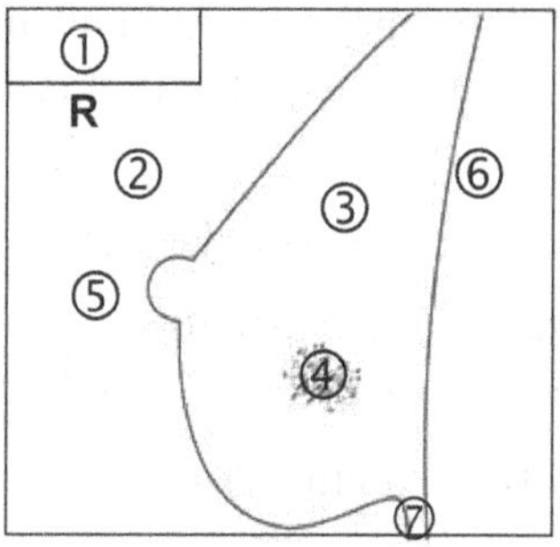

1. Identification and date.
2. Anatomical and positional markers in axillary region.
3. Whole breast imaged.
4. Skin pores demonstrating adequate compression.
5. Nipple in profile.
6. Pectoral muscle level with nipple and at correct angle.
7. Inframammary angle.

Fig. 8.3a: MLO view (Mediolateral oblique view)

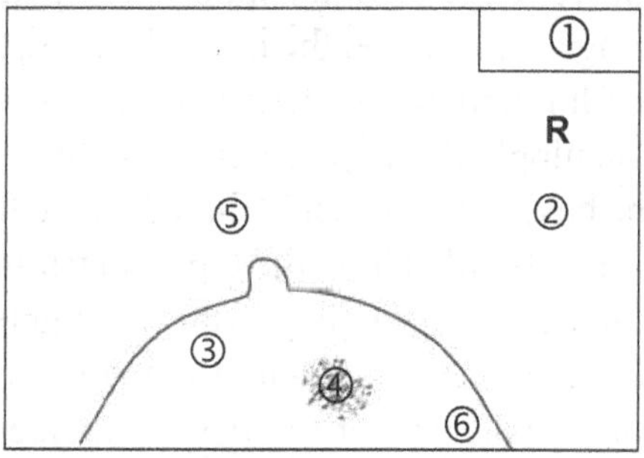

1. Identification and date.
2. Anatomical letter in axillary region.
3. Whole breast imaged demonstrating retromammary space.
4. Skin pores demonstrating adequate compression.
5. Nipple in profile.
6. Correct exposure.

Fig. 8.3b: Craniocaudal view

MLO View

Here axillary tail, pectoral muscle and inferior portion of the breast are visualised. Most abnormalities are found in upper outer quadrant and this area is clearly demonstrated in this view.

This view was devised by Lundgren and Jacobson (1976) and is universally accepted as the standard view.

Smaller the breast the steeper the angle required. The angle used should be recorded and reproduced for followup studies.

Cassette size : 18 × 24 cm or
24 × 30 cm

The patient stands facing the machine with the breast to be imaged in front of the film support. The patient stands with her feet apart to obtain a broader base and the radiographer stands directly behind the patient's back. The radiographer places her straight arm against the patient's rib cage of the side to be imaged and arm is extended forward until the fingertips touches the front of the film support ensuring that the whole body is approximately 15-18 cm away from the lower edge of film support. The patient's hand of the side to be image is placed on the head elevating the breast and the height of the film support is no less than 2 cm below the head of the humerus. The nipple lies approximately a third of the way up the film, with the base of the breast included on the film. The hand is then placed to rest tightly along the top of machine. The patient is asked to relax and not to hold tightly as this will tighten the pectoral muscle and prevent the correct angle being achieved. The radiographer stands at the patient's opposite shoulder with her foot placed against the patient's foot of the side being imaged to prevent any movement of the patient. One hand is placed against the ribs gently to push the breast forward medially towards the other hand so that the breast can be lifted and supported using the index finger and the thumb. The index finger holds the breast at the outer quadrant with the remaining fingers on the ribs and the thumb on the medial aspect at the sternum lifting and pushing the breast forward.

In this position gravity and the natural mobility of the breast pulls the tissue and pectoral muscle forward.

The radiographer places one hand in the patient's axilla with the thumb on the top of shoulder and the fingertips holding out the posterior skin folds. The patient's shoulder is lifted to create tension of skin as the breast is supported in the other hand and mid axillary skin folds prevented. While maintaining the close proximity the patient is supported and rotated 5-10° away from the film support. The patient's shoulder is raised to lift and extended the axillary area over the film. The breast is placed in and across the film with the fingers touching the upper corner of the film support so that the film is placed behind the pectoral muscle and in front of the posterior skin folds and latissimus dorsi muscle. The radiographer's elbow and forearm is used to tilt the patient's body from the waist when being moved over into position. The patient's opposite hand can be raised and placed, on the tube head temporarily to maintain balance and avoid movement if required.

Radiographer moves to behind the film support and the fingertips of the both hands are placed in the axilla to hold the anterior and posterior skin folds. The thumbs are placed on top of the shoulder joint to lift up and stretch the axillary area across the film support preventing skin folds being trapped. The radiographer stands at the opposite side of the patient with one hand under the breast and other hand under the rib so that the long part the chest is gently lifted away from the film support, without the axillary area being disturbed. The fingers should meet as the breast is lifted up and brought a little further forward and any skin folds trapped are released. The position of the breast is checked so that it lies lateral with the nipple in profile. The hand is placed underneath the breast and rotated to cup it in the palm, with the fingers spread evenly over the side and front of the breast and the thumb on the medial aspect at the sternum. The breast is held in this position with the wrist flexed to fit into inframammary angle and the elbow and forearm gently pressed into the abdomen to tilt the patient forward from the waist.

The breast is lifted upward and outwards as the opposite shoulder is rotated away slightly to avoid hurting the ribs and sternum as compression is applied. The patient is rotated back into position, once contact of the breast is made with the compression plate. The thumb and fingertips are moved forward to allow the compression plate to make contact with the breast at the chest wall, maintaining the up and out movement with the flexed wrist emphasizing the inframammary angle. When compression is complete, one hand is taken behind the patient and lifts the lower rib cage and abdomen away from the film support, to remove excess abdominal the folds. The fingers and thumb of the other hand is used to create a single fold which is pulled down so that overlap of the breast is avoided. To maintain the lift, the breast is up with the knuckles and final compression applied.

A good quality image is obtained when the axillary tail, pectoral muscle level with the nipple and at the correct angle with all the breast tissue demonstrated. When the films are viewed as mirror images, the pectoral muscle should meet and match up forming a deep 'V' with the breast matching at the inferior border.

Craniocaudal View

In this view abnormalities are seen either medial or lateral to the nipple. The patient faces the mammography machine which is in the horizontal position and the body is rotated about 15° so that the side being examined is brought close to the film support. Rotating the patient means that the film support will be in contact with the convex part of the ribs enabling the majority of the breast tissue to be demonstrated. The patient is positioned so that the nipple is in the middle of the film with the hand resting on the abdomen or on the side of the film support to relax the pectoral muscle. The patient is also encouraged to be as relaxed as possible, assuming a drooping posture with the shoulder dropped so that the breasts fall naturally forward. The radiographer stands at the opposite shoulder to the breast being imaged with the film support lower than the breast. The patient is leaned in towards the machine from the waist, and the head is rotated away from the side under examination to bring the breast closer to the film support. The breast is held with the hand in a very flat position and lifted up using the natural mobility, until it forms a right angle with chest wall. The side of the hand is placed in contact with the chest wall to avoid any loss of the posterior inferior tissue. The hand holding the breast is brought slightly forward, maintaining the lift to allow the film support to be raised until it makes contact with the breast at the junction of the inframammary angle and the chest wall. The breast is extended forward and the hand removed slowly without the breast being disturbed. The position of the nipple is checked so that it is in profile and in the midline of breast tissue. The shoulder of the side being imaged is gently pressed down to include the outer quadrant of the breast. If the shoulder is elevated, the breast is pulled up, the pectoral muscle is tightened and breast tissue will be lost. The breast is raised up off the film support with one hand while the other hand slides down the chest wall bringing in the upper posterior breast tissue. The breast is held between the hands with equal amount of inferior and posterior tissue gently stretched forward on the film support to demonstrate the maximum amount of breast tissue. The position of breast on the film support is checked so that as much as possible of the both medial and lateral aspects of the breast is included and that it is in middle of the film. The little finger and the ring finger are placed on the lateral aspect of the breast and maintaining slight pressure, the fingers are brought forward until the thumb can be placed on the medial aspect. The index and middle fingers are used then to bring down the superior posterior aspect of breast and the pectoral muscle. The position of the hand resembles the way the ball is held with the fingers spread evenly over the breast. The slight forward pressure is maintained with the finger over the breast and the patient is gently pushed with the hand on back, towards the machine preventing the natural tendency to pull away at the commencement of compression. The shoulder depressed with the hand so that the outer quadrant of the breast is brought into contact with the film support and compression is applied slowly. When the compression plate makes contact with the breast at the chest wall margin, the fingers are gradually brought forward towards the nipple maintaining the forward pull until compression is completed. After compression the patient is slightly rotated in so that the medial aspect is included. The patient gently presses the other breast in against her body to avoid skin overlapping the breast being imaged. Any skin folds at the lateral aspect are removed after compression is completed by being gently eased out using the fingertips without the breast tissue being disturbed or pulled out.

A good quality image is obtained when the maximum amount of tissue both medial and lateral aspect of the breast is demonstrated, together with the retromammary space behind the fibroglandular tissue and some pectoral muscles included.

For rest of positions for mammographic study, the readers are advised to study the *'Textbook of Mammography'*.

9

BONE DENSITY MEASUREMENT IN OSTEOPOROSIS AND OSTEOPENIA ON DEXA MACHINE

Bone density or bone mineral density (BMD) is the amount of bone mineral in bone tissue. Bone density measurement is used in clinical medicine as an indirect indicator of osteoporosis and fracture risk.

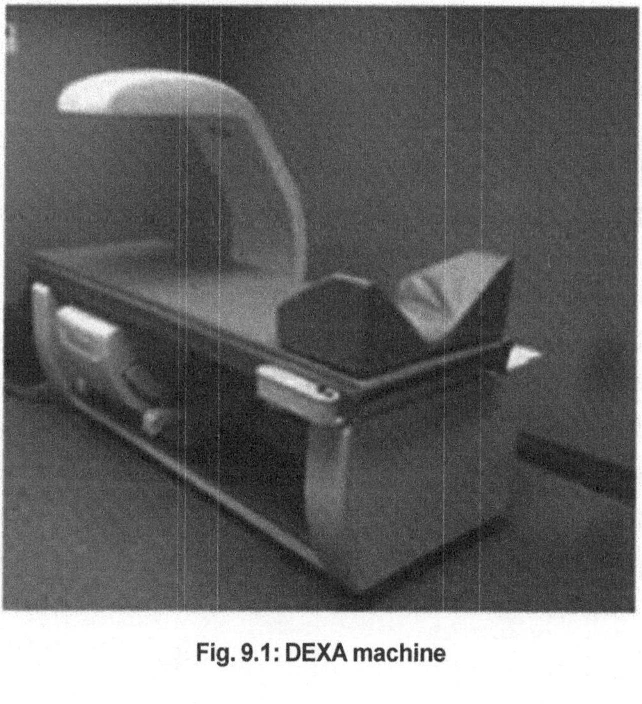

Fig. 9.1: DEXA machine

It is measured by a procedure called densitometry, often performed in the radiology or nuclear medicine department of hospitals or clinics. The measurement is painless and non-invasive and involves low radiation exposure. Measurements are most commonly made over the lumbar spine, upper part of the hip and forearm.

Fractures of the legs and pelvis due to falls are a significant public health problem, especially in elderly women, leading to much medical cost, inability to live independently and even risk of death. Bone density measurements are used to screen people for osteoporosis risk and to identify those who might benefit from measures to improve bone strength.

Indications for Testing:

- Females age 65 or older.
- Males age 70 or older.
- People over age 50 with any one of the following:
  - Previous bone fracture from minor trauma.
  - Rheumatoid arthritis.
  - Low body weight.
  - A patient with a hip fracture.
- Individuals with vertebral abnormalities.
- Individuals receiving, or planning to receive, long-term glucocorticoid (steroid) therapy.
- Individuals with primary hyperparathyroidism.
- Individuals being monitored to assess the response or efficacy of an approved osteoporosis drug therapy.
- Individuals with a history of eating disorders.
- Smoking habits.
- Drinking habit of alcohol.
- Vitamin – D deficiency.

There are many different types of BMD tests, all are non-invasive. Most tests differ according to which bones are measured to determine the BMD result.

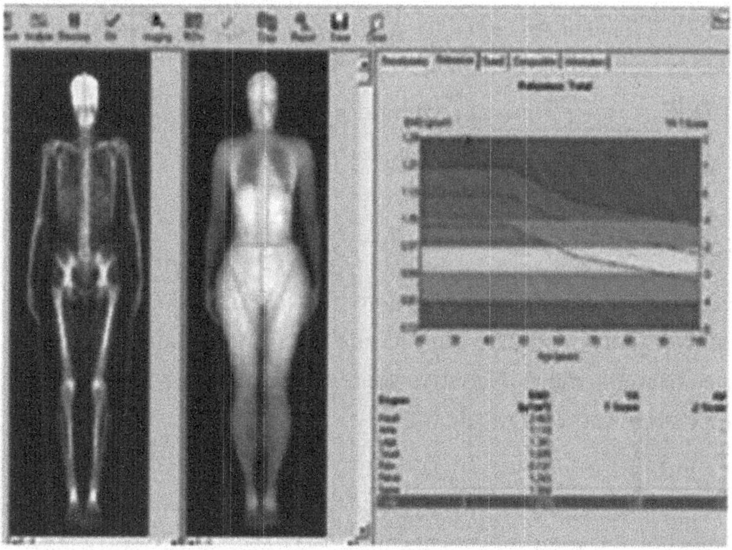

Fig. 9.2: DEXA result

These tests include:

- Dual – energy X-ray absorptiometry (DXA or DEXA).
- Dual X-ray absorptiometry and Laser (DXL).
- Quantitative computed tomography (QCT).
- Quantitative ultrasound (QUS).
- Single photon absorptiometry (SPA).
- Dual photon absorptiometry (DPA).
- Digital X-ray radiogrammetry (DXR).
- Single energy X-ray absorptiometry (SEXA).

DEXA is currently the most widely used, but quantitative ultrasound (QUS) has been described as a more cost-effective approach to measure bone density. The DEXA test works by measuring a specific bone or bones, usually the spine, hip and wrist.

The density of these bones is then compared with an average index based on age, sex and size. The resulting comparison is used to determine risk for fracture and the stage of osteoporosis (if any) in an individual.

Average bone mineral density = BMC/W [g/cm^2].

- BMC = Bone mineral content = g/cm.
- W = width at the scanned line.

Interpretation:

Results are generally scored by two measures, the T-score and the Z-score. Scores indicate the amount one's bone mineral density varies from the mean. Negative scores indicate lower bone density, and positive scores indicate higher.

T-Score:

The T-score is the relevant measure when screening for osteoporosis. It is the bone mineral density (BMD) at the site when compared to the young normal reference mean. It is a comparison of a patient's BMD to that of a healthy 30 years old.

The US standard is to use data for a 30 years old of the same sex and ethnicity, but WHO recommends using data for a 30 year old white female for everyone. Values for 30 years olds are used in post–menopausal women and men over age 50 because they better predict risk of future fracture. The criteria of the World Health Organization are:

- Normal is a T-score of –1.0 or higher.
- Osteopenia is defined as between –1.0 and –2.5.
- Osteoporosis is defined as -2.5 or lower, meaning a bone density that is two and a half standard deviations below the mean of a 30 years old man/woman.

Hip fractures per 1000 patient – year			
WHO category	**Age 50 – 64**	**Age > 64**	**Overall**
Normal	5.3	9.4	6.6
Osteopenia	11.4	19.61	5.7
Osteoporosis	22.4	46.6	40.6

Z-Score:

The Z-score is the comparison to the **age-matched normal** and is usually used in cases of severe osteoporosis. This is the number of standard deviations a patient's BMD differs from the average BMD of their age, sex and ethnicity. This value is used in premenopausal women, men under the age of 50, and in children. It is most useful when the score is less than 2 standard deviations below this normal. In this setting, it is helpful to scrutinize for coexisting illnesses or treatments that may contribute to osteoporosis such as glucocorticoid therapy, hyperparathyroidism, or alcoholism.

Limitations:

1. Measurement can be affected by the size of the patient, the thickness of tissue overlying the bone and other factors extraneous to the bones.
2. Bone density is a proxy measurement for bone strength, which is the resistance to fracture and the truly significant characteristic. Although the two are usually related, there are some circumstances in which bone density is a poorer indicator of bone strength.
3. Reference standards for some populations (e.g. children) are unavailable for many of the methods used.
4. Crushed vertebrae can result in falsely high bone density, so they must be excluded from analysis.

10

DIGITAL SUBTRACTION ANGIOGRAPHY

Acquisition of digital fluoroscopic images combined with injection of contrast media and real time subtraction of pre and post contrast images to perform angiography is referred to as digital subtraction angiography.

It is used oftenly in interventional radiology for very clear visualization of blood vessels in a bony or dense tissue environment.

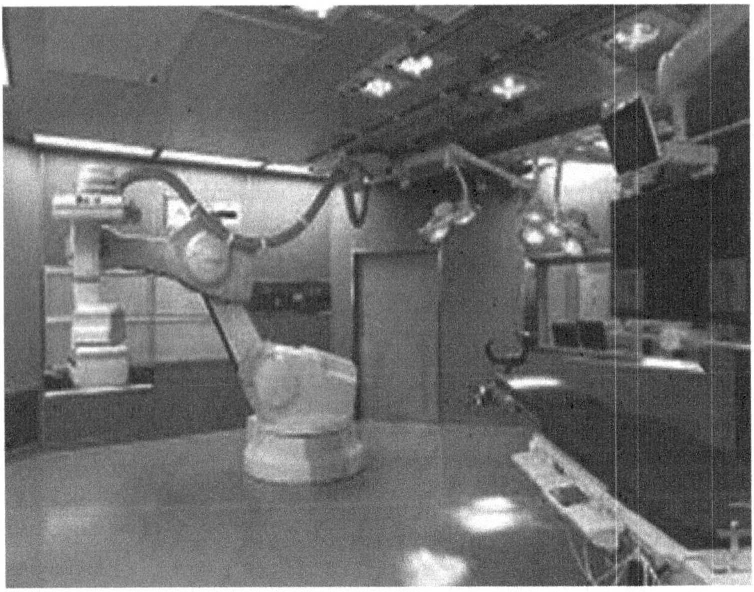

Fig. 10.1: Digital subtraction angiography machine

Indication:

1. Cerebrovascular anatomy.
2. Common carotid artery.
3. Internal carotid artery and its branches i.e. anterior, middle cerebral arteries.
4. External carotid artery and its branches i.e. superior thyroid, ascending pharyngeal, occipital, superficial temporal, maxillary facial, lingual and middle meningeal arteries.

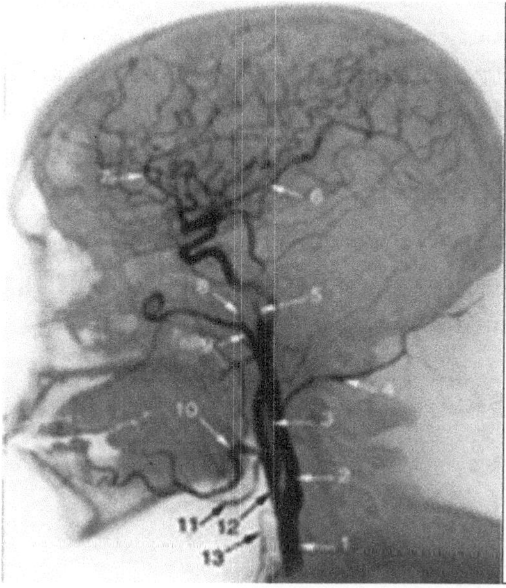

Identification
1. Common carotid artery.
2. Internal carotid artery.
3. Ascending pharyngeal artery.
4. Occipital artery.
5. Superficial temporal artery.
6. Middle cerebral artery.
7. Anterior cerebral artery.
8. Middle meningeal artery.
9. Maxillary artery.
10. Facial artery.
11. Lingual artery.
12. External carotid artery.
13. Superior thyroid artery.

Fig. 10.2: Cerebral angiography on DSA

"Angio" means blood vessel and angiography is the radiological study of blood vessel in the body after administration of iodinated contrast media.

"Subtraction" word is simply a technique by which bone structural images are subtracted or cancelled out from a film of bones plus opacified vessels, leaving an unobscured image of the vessels alone.

Procedure:

- Gaining arterial access.
- Selective arterial catheterization.
- Image acquisition.
- Closure of arterial access.
- Post processing.
- Hard copy.

Principle:

- Blood vessels are not normally seen on an X-ray image because of low contrast, but better seen in D.S.A.
- Dense fluid with high atomic numbers increase the contrast e.g. iodine.
- Iodine absorbs photons more than blood and tissue.
- The first contrast media used for intravascular injection "**High osmolar contrast media**".

Advantage of CO_2DSA:

- Non-allergic.
- Non-nephrotoxic.
- Can use unlimited total volumes.
- Low viscosity (1/400 that of contrast).
  - Improves detection of acute hemorrhage.
  - May enhance demonstration of AV fissula, tumor vessels.
  - Easier demonstration through micro catheter.
  - Can be administered around wire in catheter using a Y–connector without losing wire position.
  - Portal vein opacification.
  - Can be administered via superfine small needles (25-27

gauge) with less invasiveness.
 - Central reflux.
 - Can demonstrate entire vessels, central and parietal to catheter end hole unlike contrast.
- Not diluted by blood like contrast.
- Inexpensive (100 cc/volume is required).
- Primarily for vasculature, can also be used in any luminal structure, e.g., biliary ducts.

DSA could be:

1. Intra-arterial DSA.
2. Intravenous DSA–is a computer technique which compares an X-ray image of a region of body before and after radiopaque iodine based dye has been injected intravenously into the body. Tissues and blood vessels on first image are digitally subtracted from second image, leaving a clean picture of the artery which can then be studied independently and in isolation from the rest of body.

   Not suitable for patient with diabetes or renal insufficiency because dye load is significantly higher than that used in arteriorgraphy.

   Helpful in carotid artery obstruction and to study cerebral blood flow. It helps detect and diagnose lesions in the carotid arteries, a potential cause of strok.

   Can assess patients prior to surgery, after coronary artery bypass surgery and transplant patient.

11

Harmful Effects of Radiation

X-rays are only dangerous and harmful if you are careless.

Care means adhering to the following rules:

- Stand behind the control panel when X-ray exposure is made.
- Make sure that lead aprons and lead gloves are worn if the patient needs to be held.
- If possible, do not allow any one else in the X-ray room. If other persons must be present, keep them behind the control panel when the exposure is made.
- Wear your film badge always. Have it checked regularly.
- Never take an X-ray unless ordered by a doctor or other qualified medical person.

X-ray may cause harm. You cannot feel or see them. You may not know, you are in the X-ray beam, put repeated exposure to X-rays, even those that are scattered off the patient or the X-ray equipment, and even in small doses, can cause permanent damage to the health of the X-ray operator or anyone else. Remember again, it is not only the direct beam of X-rays that may be harmful, but also the scattered rays.

You must never make an X-ray exposure when you are anywhere near the X-ray tube; you must always be behind the control panel and there you are safe.

You must not allow any one except the patient to be in the X-ray room, unless the patient needs to be supported or a child needs to be held. When that is necessary, the parent or friend must wear a lead apron and lead gloves whenever he or she is near the patient while the X-ray is being taken. Do not let a nurse or any other member of the hospital staff hold a patient while an exposure is being made.

The risk for patients being X-rayed is very low because they are exposed to X-rays infrequently, and only a small part of body is exposed for each picture. But try to get all the details right before taking the first time so that there is no need for a second exposure.

The greatest risk from X-rays is for the operator, the doctor and the nurses, who may be exposed repeatedly over the years while they are working.

RADIATION MEASUREMENTS AND ITS BIOLOGICAL EFFECTS

INTRODUCTION

Radiation measurement units have undergone a change from Rads and Rems to Grays and Sieverts. Radiation exposure is quantified by the unit Kerma which is now expressed in Grays and Sieverts.

Radiation Definition and Properties

Radiation is defined as energy in transit and comprises electromagnetic rays (X-rays or gamma rays) and particulate radiation (electrons, protons, neutrons, alpha particles, negative pimesons, and heavily charged ions). X-rays and gamma rays are identical except that they differ only in their source of origin. X-rays are produced mechanically by making electrons strike a target that cause the electrons to give up their energy as X-rays, whereas gamma rays produced by nuclear disintegration of radioactive isotopes.(Cho *et al.*, 1998)

X-rays and gamma rays are packets of energy or photons and have no mass or charge. They travel in straight lines. The wavelength of X-rays is 10^{-10} meters which is 1A° (A°= angstrom).

The wavelength, λ of electromagnetic radiation is related to the frequency ν by the formula:

$\lambda\nu = c$ (where c is the speed of light)

Wavelength being inversely proportional to frequency, can also be denoted as $\omega = c/\lambda$.

Each photon contains energy equal to hn,

or $E = h\nu$ (where h is Plank's constant, Plank's constant = 6.634×10^{-34})

Since $\lambda n = c$ and $n = c/\lambda$,

The energy of X-rays can be calculated, by replacing n in the equation $E = hn$

as $E = hc/\lambda$

The difference between non-ionizing and ionizing radiation is the energy of the individual photons and is not dependent on the energy of the total dose of radiation.

Units of Radiation and Exposure

The unit of radiation exposure is the Roentgen (R) defined as an amount of X-rays or gamma rays that produces a specific amount of ionization in a unit of air under standard temperature and pressure; this quantity can be measured directly in an air chamber. It is 2.58×10^{-4} C/kg air.[Brateman L, 1999] Exposure is defined strictly for air as the interacting medium.

Exposure is quantified by the unit Kerma. Kerma is an acronym for kinetic energy released in material. Kerma quantifies the amount of energy transferred to charged particles from ionizing photon radiation. The unit of Kerma was the Rad and is now the Gray (Gy). The unit for measurement of the amount of energy deposited in tissue is the 'rad' or radiation absorbed dose.

The unit rad is defined as the absorption of 0.01 joule of energy in one kg of material. This unit is now replaced by Gray. One Gray is the absorption of one joule per kg of tissue (i.e., one gray = 100 rads).

Since 1 rad = 0.01 joule energy/kg

and 1 Gray = 1 joule per kg

Therefore, 1 Gray = 100 rads.

For air, 1 Gy of Kerma is equivalent to 115R of exposure, which has been rounded off 1 cGy being approximately = 1 Roentgen.(Brateman L, 1999)

When X-rays are absorbed in tissue, energy may break chemical bonds and thus cause damage to the cells that comprise the tissue. The biological effectiveness of a given absorbed dose of one type of ionizing radiation is not necessarily the same as that of an equally absorbed dose of another type of radiation. For this reason, a unit of radiation dose equivalent was developed which was called, 'rem', and acronym for Roentgen equivalent man. It represents dose in rads multiplied by a quality factor, QF (also called relative biological effectiveness, RBE). The quality factor for the various types of radiations is as follows: (Campeau FE, 1999)

Sl.No.	*Type of Radiation*	*Quality factor*
1.	X, gamma or beta radiation	1
2.	Alpha particles and multiple charged particles	20
3.	Neutrons	10
4.	High energy protons	10

The radiation dose equivalent for which the unit was rem, has now been replaced by 'Sievert' in the SI units.

Sievert is defined as the dose in Gray multiplied by the quality factor. The Sievert is currently used for devising radiation protection standards (Sv = Gray × QF).

Kerma	=	Kinetic Energy transferred to changed particles in Rads/Gray
Rad	=	Radiation absorbed dose

	=	100 ergs of energy/gm of tissue
	=	0.01 joule of energy/kg of tissue
1 Gray	=	100 Rads = 1 joule of energy/kg of tissue
1 Rad	=	0.01 Gray
1 cGy (centi Gray)	=	1 Rad
1 mGy (milli Gray)	=	0.1 Rad
Rem	=	Radiation equivalent man
	=	Rad × RBE (QF)/(relative biological effectiveness or Quality factor)
Sievert	=	Gray × QF
1 Sievert	=	100 rems
(1000 milli Sv or mSv)		
1 mSv	=	0.1 rem (for X-rays which have a qualifying factor of 1) = 1 mGy

The DS-86 System

The radiation exposure by atomic bomb is currently measured by a dosimetry system devised in 1986, and is called the DS-86 system. This system follows the current units of Grays and Sieverts and is used for calculating the organ doses. DS-86 system takes into account the spectrum and amount of radiation released by the bombs, attenuation with distance and physical shielding, free in air Kerma reaching the person, body position with respect to atom bomb position, and also the further attenuation of the radiation reaching the gonads by the intervening body tissues.[Neel *et al.*, 1990]

Sources of Radiation

The natural sources include cosmic radiation from space, radiation from the earth and its internal radionulides. Artificial sources of radiation include X-ray equipment, nuclear weapons and radioactive medication.

Most of a person's lifetime radiation exposure is from low dose background radiation. The average annual effective dose for persons in the United States is estimated to be about 3.6 mSv. About two-thirds of this radiation is from natural sources, of which radon, cosmic rays, radionucleides in the earth and radioactive elements in the body are the major contributors. Radon is believed to contribute about 55 percent of a person's total background radiation exposure. This represents about 2 mSv of exposure per year. Radon is a colorless, odorless and tasteless alpha particle emitting radioactive gas, which is derived from naturally occurring uranium deposits in the earth. Radon itself is not particularly harmful, but some of its alpha-elements polonium radioactive decay products may heavily irradiate bronchial epithelium cells for many months or years.

Cosmic radiation accounts for about 0.3 mSv of background radiation per year at sea level. The earth's atmosphere acts as a shield, so that the dose is about doubled with every 1500 meters increase in altitude. Radioactive potassium and carbon and other radionuclides within the body contribute about another 0.4 mSv to the average person's annual background radiation exposure. Radioactive decay of thorium and uranium radionuclides in the earth's crust constitute the major sources of terrestrial radiation, which, in most areas, is about 0.3 mSv per year. The remaining 18 percent of a person's total background radiation exposure is from man-made sources. Diagnostic X-ray and nuclear medicine account for over 0.5 mSv of the estimated annual total of about 0.65 mSv.

Effects of Radiation

For effects of radiation see Flowchart 11.1.

Historical Aspects

Discovery of X-rays by Roentgen on 8th November, 1895. Within few months of Roentgen's discovery, eye complaints and severe progressive dermatitis were reported. In 1896, Clearance E Dally developed ulcerating carcinoma. Delayed effects of radiation began

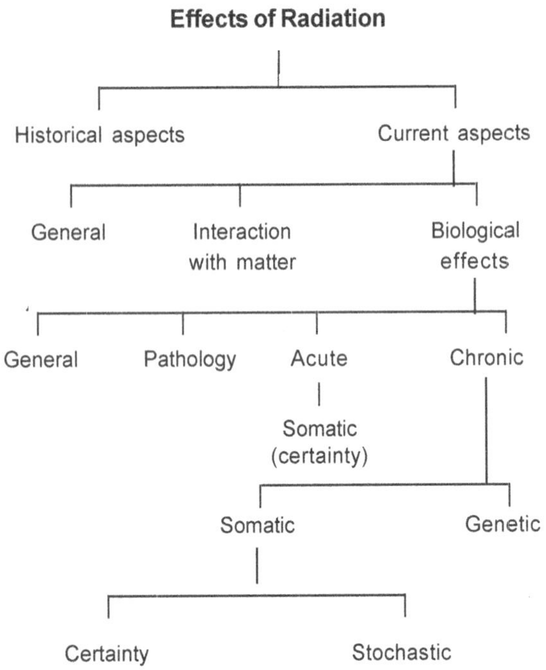

Flowchart 11.1

to be documented only 20 years after their initial discovery. Germ line mutation as a delayed effect of ionizing radiation was documented by Müller in 1927 who was awarded Nobel prize. In 1936, Percy Brown a Radiologist historian, recorded case histories of adverse effects of radiation which occurred in people exposed from 1911 onwards. In 1942, Dunlap reported radiation induced leukemia in Radiologists and other radiation workers.(Miller RW, 1995)

Current Concepts of Radiation Hazards

General

In the current context, it is believed that without proper precautions radiation sources are just as dangerous as they were earlier.

In India, we are in a scenario of two groups of people, one with complete ignorance of radiation hazards, which comprise a vast majority and the other a small minority of educated patients who are terrified of even tiny radiation exposures. The latter group being more common in developed countries, are more sensitized and have even launched litigation suits against companies producing radioactive materials.

Interaction of Radiation with Matter

There are three major ways in which radiation, especially X-rays is absorbed and results in ionization: the photoelectric effect, the Compton effect and pair production. At low energies (30 to 100 kev), as in diagnostic radiology, the photoelectric effect is important. In this process, the incident photon interacts with an electron in one of the outer shells of an atom (typically K, L or M). If the energy of the photon is greater than the binding energy of the electron, then the electron is expelled from the orbit with a kinetic energy that is equal to the energy of the incident photon minus the binding energy of the electron. The photoelectric effect varies as a function of the cube of the atomic number of the material exposed (z) this fact explains why bone is visualized much better than soft tissue on radiograph.(Cho *et al.*, 1998)

Biological Effects of Radiation

General Principles

1. The interaction of radiation in a cell is a probably function or a matter of change, i.e., an interaction may or may not occur. Furthermore, the occurrence of an interaction does not necessarily mean that damage will result. In fact, damage is frequently repaired.
2. The initial deposition of energy occurs very rapidly, within 10^{-18} seconds.
3. Radiation deposits energy in a cell in a random fashion.
4. Radiation produces no unique changes in cells, tissues or organs. The changes induced by radiation are indistinguishable from

damage produced by other types of trauma.

5. The biological changes in cells, tissues, and organs do not appear immediately. They occur only after a period of time (latent period), ranging from hours (e.g., after accidental overexposures to the total body, resulting in failure of organ system and death), to as long as years (e.g., in the case of radiation-induced cancer) or even generations (such as is the case if the damage occurs in a germ cell leading to heritable changes). The length of the latency period depends on factors related to the radiation, basically of radiation exposure, the dose as well as to biological characteristics of the cell irradiated and most importantly their rate of division and to the frequency of their rate of division.(Travis E, 1997)

Radiation may deposit energy directly within the critical target of the cell, which is the DNA; this type of action is known as the direct action. Biological effects of radiation including cell killing, mutagenesis and carcinogenesis are all due to damage to DNA, i.e., the direct action. Interaction of radiation with the other molecules in the cell is an indirect action. Indirect action is due to action on the major constituents of the cell, which are the water molecules. Radiation releases OH ions from water molecules, which cause the cell damage due to their oxidizing effect.

Mean Lethal Dose or LD50: The lethal dose 50 or LD50 is defined as the dose of an agent that causes mortality in 50% of given population in a given time. Humans can survive a total body dose of 4 Gy, estimates of LD50 for a human is 3 to 4 Gy. (Travis E, 1997)

Pathology of Radiation Injury

Irradiated cells die either a mitotic death which is also called reproductive failure. Mitotic death occurs when an irradiated cell attempts to undergo mitosis. Mitotic death can occur after relatively small doses of radiation. The other form of death is apoptosis or programmed cell death. Apoptosis is a natural form of cell death, which occurs spontaneously without a cytotoxic insult.

Acute responses to radiation therapy are seen in tissues with rapid turnover (gastrointestinal mucosa, bone marrow, skin, oropharyngeal and esophageal mucosa). Acute radiation damage leads to cell necrosis. In chronic radiation injury, atrophy, necrosis, ulceration, metaplasia, dysplasia or neoplasia can occur in epithelial and parenchymal cells. In the stromal tissue, changes that are seen are: fibrosis, necrosis and presence of atypical fibroblasts. Arteries and capillaries show endothelial cell damage, thrombosis, rupture, myointimal proliferation and vasculitis. Small veins show intimal proliferation, fibrosis and veno occlusive disease as in the liver.(Fazardo IGLF, 1998)

CLASSIFICATION OF RADIATION INJURY

Radiation effects are classified as: Acute or chronic, involving somatic tissues or genetic information, and be directly proportional to dose, i.e., deterministic (certainty) effects, or not directly proportional to dose, i.e., stochastic effects.

1. **Somatic**
   a. *Certainty or deterministic effects*
      - Related with certainty to a known dose of radiation.
      - Dose threshold exists.
      - Severity is dose related.

   b. *Stochastic effects*
      - Random events without threshold.
      - Probability increases with dose.
      - Severity may not be dose related.
2. **Genetic**—Are stochastic by their nature.

Deterministic effects as documented from radiation accidents and from patients undergoing radiotherapy:

Acute Total Body Irradiation: At doses in excess of 100 Gy to the total body, death usually occurs within 24 and 48 hours from neurologic and cardiovascular failure. This is known as the cerebrovascular syndrome. Because cerebrovascular damage cause death very quickly, the failure of other systems do not have time to develop. At doses between 5 and 12 Gy, death may occur in a matter of days, as a result of the gastrointestinal syndrome. The symptoms during this period may include nausea, vomiting and prolonged diarrhoea, for several days, leading to dehydration, sepsis and death.

At total body doses between 2 and 8 Gy, death may occur several weeks after exposure and is due to effects on the bone marrow, which results in the hemopoietic syndrome. The full effect of radiation is not apparent until the mature hematopoietic cells are depleted. Death from the hematologic damage occurs at about 20 to 30 days after exposure and the risk of death continues over the next 30 days. Clinical symptoms during this period may include chills, fatigue and petechial hemorrhage. The threshold for this syndrome is 1 Gy. At Chernobyl, approximately 200 employees were exposed to radiation >1 Gy and exhibited overt signs of the hemopoietic syndrome.

Chronic Radiation Effects: These effects result from prolonged exposure of lower intensity or may appear as late effects in survivors of more acute exposures. These may be due to whole body or partial body irradiation.

Somatic Certainty Effects on Organ Systems (as evaluated in patients on radiotherapy): Somatic Certainty Effects:

Central Nervous System: Central nervous system (CNS) has been described as relatively resistant to radiation-induced changes. When the human brain is treated with standard fractionation (1.8 to 2.0 Gy/d), acute reactions are seldom observed. Subacute CNS reactions to radiation treatment are more common. Mild encephalopathy and focal neurologic changes can occur after irradiation limited to the cranium. The effect of cranial irradiation is believed to be secondary to radiation effects on the replicating oligodendrocytes and possibly on the microvasculature. Post-irradiation pathology and associated clinical symptoms typically begin

6 to 36 months after radiation therapy. A unique late effect of cranial irradiation combined with chemotherapy, known as leukoencephalopathy, has been described as a necrotizing reaction usually noted 4 to 12 months after combined treatment with methotrexate and cranial irradiation. Radiation necrosis occurs in 1% to 5% of patients after 55 to 60 gray doses, fractionated over 6 weeks; 75% of cases occur within 3 years.(Rubin *et al.*, 1998)

Transverse myelitis after radiation treatment is a spinal cord reaction similar to cerebral necrosis. This syndrome consists of progressive and irreversible leg weakness and loss of bladder function and sensation referable to a single spinal cord level. Flaccid paralysis eventually occurs. Symptoms can occur as early as 6 months after radiation treatment, but the usual time to onset is 12 to 24 months. Marcus and Million showed that at 45 Gy, the incidence of radiation myelitis is <0.2%.

Skin: Skin reaction can be seen within 2 weeks of fractionated radiotherapy, a delay that correlates with the time required for cells to move from the basal to the keratinized layer of skin. Erythema is observed soon followed by dry desquamation.

A chronic reaction to radiation can be seen starting 6 to 12 months after irradiation. The epidermis is usually atrophic and it may be more easily injured than normal skin. The amount of interstitial fibrosis may also be increased. Hyperpigmentation of irradiated skin outlining the treatment field can be seen within a couple of months after completion of irradiation. The skin becomes thin and hair loss may be permanent.(Cho *et al.*, 1998)

Heart and Blood Vessels: Acute "pericarditis" may result from cardiac irradiation. Symptoms may include chest pain and fever, with or without pericardial effusion. Asymptomatic pericardial effusion may be common presentation. Constructive pericarditis occurs as a result of more than 40 Gy to a large portion of the heart. Chronic cardiac changes from 6 months to several years after irradiation.

Lung: Pneumonitis may appear within 3 to 6 weeks if a large region of lung is irradiated to a dose above 25 Gy. An infiltrate outlining the treatment field may become evident on the chest X-ray. At 8.2 Gy, there is a 5% incidence of lethal radiation induced pneumonitis which increases to 80% at 11 Gray.

Digestive Tract: The mucosa of the GI tract is a rapid renewal system, with dramatic mucosal changes appearing within 7 to 14 days. Nausea and vomiting, diarrhoea and cramping pain are usual presentations. Factors contributing to the pathogenesis of diarrhoea include malabsorption and alterations in the intestinal bacterial flora. Chronic radiation enteropathy include diarrhoea, abdominal cramp, nausea, malabsorption, vomiting and obstruction. Progressive fibrosis, perforation, fistula formation and stenosis of the irradiated portion of the bowel can also occur during the chronic phase of radiation enteropathy. Most clinical manifestations of chronic changes occur between 6 months and 5 years after radiation therapy.

Hemopoietic system: Fractionated radiation to a localized area of the marrow to a unique lesion of adipose tissue replacing the marrow, instead of fibrotic tissue occurs in other organs. This change is recorded at a threshold dose greater than 50 Gy.

Eye: Cataract has been recorded at 2-8 Gray of single exposure.(Rubin *et al.*, 1998)

Bladder: Radiation injury to the bladder generally becomes symptomatic 3 to 6 weeks after the start of treatment and symptoms usually subside 3 to 4 weeks after completion of radiation therapy. Cystoscopy often shows diffuse mucosal changes similar to those of acute cystitis. The late effects of high radiation doses to the bladder may include interstitial fibrosis, telangiectasia and ulceration. A contracted bladder may result from doses in excess of 60 Gy. (Cho *et al.*, 1998)

Testis and Ovaries: Type B spermatogonia are sensitive to the effects of radiation. Type A spermatogonia are thought to be more resistant because their longer cell cycle time allows considerable variation in radiosensitivity among different phases of the cell cycle. Sertoli cells and Leydig cells are less radiosensitive than the spermatogonia. The single dose required for permanent sterilization in normal male is not clearly established but it is believed to be between 6 and 10 Gy. Low dose fractionated irradiation leads to decreases in sperm count. Regeneration of spermatogonia usually does not begin until 2 to 8 weeks after the injury.

The radiation dose necessary to induce ovarian failure is age dependent. A single dose of 3 to 4 Gy can induce amenorrhoea in almost all women over 40 years of age. In young women, oogenesis is much less sensitive to radiation than spermatogenesis is in men.(Cho *et al.*, 1998)

Tolerance doses to whole organ irradiation

Single dose (Gy)		*Fractionated dose (Gy)*	
Bone marrow	2-10	Testes	1-2
Ovary	2-6	Ovary	6-10
Testes	2-10	Eye (Lens)	6-12
Eye (Lens)	2-10	Thyroid	30-40

Somatic Stochastic Effects

These are late effects, which occur at random with no dose threshold. All stochastic effects are late but not all late effects are stochastic. The probability of their occurrence increases with increase in the absorbed dose but not their severity. The effects of shortening of life span and induction of malignancies are considered somatic stochastic effects.

Shortening of Life Span: This has been reported in laboratory mice.(Miller RW, 1995)

Leukemia: Acute and chronic myeloid leukemias may occur. During childhood, acute lymphatic leukemia occur with, latency period, minimum of 2 years.(Sinclare, 1995)

Other Radiation Induced Cancers

Malignancies of skin, lung, bone, blood dyscrasia and meningiomas have been described. Thyroid carcinomas in children living in areas with contamination from the Chernobyl accident.

Risk Estimates for Radiation Induced Cancer

The likelihood of developing radiation induced cancer is described as a "cancer risk".

Absolute Risk: Risk increases for a period of time and then decreases, an example of this type of cancer risk is radiation induced leukemia.

Relative Risk: Risk increased by a constant factor for all ages.

Mechanism of Radiation Induced Cancer

There are 3 potential mechanisms, basically genetic in nature. Check point genes that control cellular proliferation and differentiation may be disrupted, activation of oncogenes may occur, loss of suppressor genes may induce cancer. Genetic mechanism of radiation induces cancers. DNA and chromosomal changes can give rise to malignancies either by activation of oncogenes or by the loss of suppressor genes. Oncogenes are mutated genes that are thought to be involved in the transformation of a normal cell to a malignant phenotype. Radiation can activate oncogenes through a number of mechanisms including point mutation, chromosomal rearrangement of chromosomal translocations. Suppressor genes may also be involved in the change to a malignant phenotype via a chromosomal aberration.

Genetic Effects of Radiation

Radiation can either damage the DNA or effect the chromosome itself. Genetic effects on human manifests as mutations leading to congenital defects in the offspring or causing malignancies.

Mutational effects is expressed as the "genetic doubling dose". Genetic doubling dose is an estimate of the amount of acute radiation which will double the spontaneous mutation rate or will cause an increase in the mutation rate which is equal to the number of spontaneous mutations which normally occur. The most common genetic effects such as autosomal and X-linked changes and chromosome alterations in an exposed population have been estimated to be occurring at 1×10^{-2} Sv^{-1} (0.01 mutations per Sv).

Pathophysiology of Genetic Effects of Radiation

1. *Radiation Damage to DNA*

DNA is a critical target for radiation. DNA consists of two strands that form a double helix. The backbone of each strand is made up of sugar moieties and phosphate groups, which serve as the framework for the four bases. The order of these bases on the sugar-phosphate backbone spells out the genetic code.

Radiation can damage either the backbone of DNA, producing strand breaks, or it can produce alterations or loss of bases. Strand breaks may occur in only one of the strands or in both strands. SSBs are more readily required. DSBs particularly if they are repaired at a slower rate than SSBs. DSBs are known to be correlated with higher rate of cell death, as compared to SSBs. Ataxia telangiectasia is a rare genetic disorder associated with deficiency of DNA repair.

2. *Chromosomal Effects*

Radiation produces breaks in chromosomes, termed aberrations.

The general consequences of these breaks are as follows:

- The ends of the same chromosome may rejoin, a process called restitution. This causes no change.
- The sticky end of one chromosome may join with that of

another, leading to reassortment of the genetic material and an aberration visible at the net metaphase.

- The broken ends may not rejoin. The genetic material contained in the acentric fragment will be lost from the cell.

Loss of a significant amount of genetic material results in cell death, loss of a lesser amount of genetic material is a "deletion". Chromosomal aberrations are associated with certain malignancies: Burkitt's lymphoma, acute promyelocytic leukemia and ovarian cancer. Tumors associated with deletions include small cell lung cancer, neuroblastoma, retinoblastoma and Wilms' tumor.

Effects on the Fetus May be Both Deterministic and Stochastic

Deterministic Effects on the Fetus

Deterministic effects result from the killing of cells and there is a threshold dose. Examples are fetal death, gross malformations, mental retardation and growth retardation. CNS malformations are encephaly, microcephaly, mental retardation, skull malformations and hydrocephaly. The ocular malformations reported with radiation are absence of eyes, microphthalmia, absence of lens and cataract. Skeletal malformations are stunting, cleft palpate, club feet, deformed arms and spina bifida. Other malformations are genital deformities.

Effects of Radiation on Various Stages of the Fetus

Radiation during the pre-implantation period can lead to death of the embryo and the incidence is 6.9% with a dose of 0.5 Gy. During 9-60 days post conception, at a threshold dose of 10 cG the incidence dose of 10 cGy the incidence of fetal mortality is 4.8% and the risk of malformation is 0.5% per cGy. At 61-104 days post-conception the threshold for lethality is 0.5 Gy and radiation at this stage leads to either to fetal death or to brain malformations.

Estimated fetal exposure for various diagnostic imaging methods

Examination type	*Estimated fetal dose per examination (rad)**	*Estimated fetal dose per examination (m gray/m Sv)**	*Number of examinations required for a cumulative 5-rad (0.05 gray) dose*
Plain films			
Skull	0.004	0.04	1,250
Chest (two views)	0.00007	0.0007	71,429
Mammogram	0.002	0.02	250
Lumbosacral spine	0.359	3.59	13
Pelvis	0.040	0.40	125
CT scans (slice thickness: 10 mm)			
Head (10 slices)	<0.050	<0.50	>100
Abdomen (10 slices)	<0.100	<1.0	>50
Fluoroscopic studies			
Upper GI series	0.56	5.6	89
Nuclear medicine studies			
Most studies using technetium (99m Tc)	<0.500	<5.00	>10
Environmental sources			
(For comparison) Environmental background radiation (cumulative dose over nine months)	0.100	1.00	N/A

At 105-175 days post-conception the defects are mental retardation, small head size and growth retardation, at this stage the threshold for growth retardation is 0.5 Gy. At more than 175 days post-conception the risk for malformation and mental retardation are negligible.

Stochastic effects are caused by mutations in a cell or in a small group of cells.

It has been estimated that radiation doses to the order of 10 mGy received by the fetus in utero produces an increased risk of childhood leukemia at the rate of 6% per Gy.

Safety of Radiographic Imaging During Pregnancy

The effects on fetus are radiation induced teratogenesis, malignancies and genetic mutations. For mental retardation and lowering of IQ the threshold is perhaps 0.1 to 0.2 Gy and the most sensitive period is 8-17 weeks of gestation. The accepted cumulative dose of ionizing radiation during pregnancy is 5 rad (0.05 Gray or 5 m Gray or 50 mSv), and no single diagnostic study exceeds this maximum.

The Pregnant Radiation Worker

The NCRP (National Radiological Protection Board of America) recommends that the dose to the fetus in female radiation workers should not exceed 0.5 mSv per month (i.e., 0.5 mGy or 0.05 Rad per month for X-rays). The ICRP (International Council for Radiation Protection) recommends that the total dose to the abdomen of the mother should not exceed 2 mSv during entire pregnancy.(Sinclare, 1995)

Safety of Pelvimetry Techniques

MRI should be used whenever required. If CT is used, then a single lateral scanogram at the lowest mAs should be obtained whenever CT is not available, a single lateral view using an air gap technique without a grid, with good coning and fast film screen combination gives maximum information.(Thomas *et al.*, 1988)

Biological Effects of Paternal Preconception Irradiation

Paternal preconception irradiation (PPI) is not associated with an increased risk of childhood cancer. Goldstein and Murphy have reported that preconception maternal irradiation in therapeutic doses gives rise to defects in 1 out of 10 or 11 exposed children.(Steenvoorde *et al.*, 1998)

[redacted]

(ICRP), the National Commission for Radiation Protection (NCRP) in America, and the Atomic Energy Regularity Board (AERB) in India. These bodies recommend norms for permissible doses of radiation from X-ray tubes and the shielding required for the walls of an X-ray room. The duties of the Radiation Safety Officer (RSO) are also specified by the regulatory bodies, as are the radiation surveillance and radiation safety programmers.

The Regulatory Bodies

The Regulatory Bodies lay down norms for protection against radiation and also recommend the dose limits for radiation workers and the general public. The ICRP (International Commission for Radiation Protection) is the international regulatory body. Each country has its national counterpart of the ICRP. In America, the counterpart is the NCRP or The National Commission for Radiological Protection and in India it is the AERB or the Atomic Energy Regulatory Board.

The International Commission of Radiation Protection (ICRP) was formed in 1928 on the recommendation of the first International Congress of Radiology in 1925, and consists of 12 members, a chairman and a secretary. The first International Congress also initiated the birth of the ICRU or the International Commission on Radiation Units and Measurements.

The Indian Regulatory Board is the AERB (Atomic Energy Regulatory Board), constituted on November 15, 1983 by the President of India by exercising the powers conferred by section 27 of the Atomic Energy Act, 1962 (33 of 1962) to carry out certain regulatory and safety functions under the Act. The regulatory authority of AERB is derived from the rules and notifications promulgated under the Atomic Energy Act, 1962 and the Environmental (Protection) Act, 1986. The mission of the Board is to ensure that the use of ionizing radiation of the Board is to ensure the use of ionizing radiation and nuclear energy in India does not cause undue risk to health and environment.

Objectives of Radiation Protection

The ICRP in 1991 stated that "the overall objective of radiation protection is to provide an appropriate standard of protection for man without limiting the beneficial practices giving rise to radiation exposure". ICRP suggested, "current standards of protection are meant to prevent occurrence of deterministic effects by keeping doses below relevant thresholds and ensure that all reasonable steps are taken to reduce induction of stochastic effects".(Seeram *et al.*, 1997)

Radiation Safety Act in India

Radiation safety in handling of radiation generating equipment is governed by section 17 of the Atomic Energy Act, 1962, and the Radiation Protection Rules (RPR), GSR—1601, 1971 issued under the Act. The "Radiation Surveillance Procedures of Medical Applications of Radiations, GSR—388, 1989", issued under rule 15 specify general requirements for ensuring radiation protection in installation and handling of X-ray equipment. It was revised by AERB in the year 2001.

Role of AERB (India)

AERB of India recommends and lays guidelines regarding the specifications of medical X-ray equipment, for the room layout of X-ray installation, regarding the work practices in X-ray department, the protective devices and also the responsibilities of the radiation personnel, employer and Radiation Safety Officer (RSO). AERB is the authority in India which exercises a regulatory control on the approval of new models of X-ray equipment and the layout of any new proposed X-ray installation. It is also the regulatory authority for registration and commissioning of new X-ray equipment, inspection and decommissioning of X-ray installation, certification of an RSO and of service engineers and also for imposing penalties on any person contravening these rules.

Radiologists and technologists understand risks of radiation and also its advantages or benefits to the patients. Cancer induction and genetic effects are stochastic effects and cataracts, blood dyscrasia and impaired fertility are examples of deterministic effects. The benefits of diagnostic radiology in orthopedic, gastrointestinal and neurological disorders is well-known. Screening mammography in asymptomatic women below 35 years of age is considered to have a low benefit to risk ratio.

Radiation protection standards are based on three general principles:

a. Justification of a practice, i.e., no practice involving exposure to radiation should be adopted unless it provides sufficient benefit to offset the detrimental effects of radiation.

b. Protection should be optimized in relation to the magnitude of doses, number of people exposed and also to optimize it for all social and economic strata of patients.

c. Dose limitation, on the other hand, deals with the idea of establishing annual dose limits for occupational exposures, public exposures, and exposures to the embryo and fetus.

Optimization of Protection and the ALARA Principle

Optimization of protection can be achieved by optimizing the procedure to administer a radiation dose which is as low as reasonably achievable (ALARA). ALARA and ORP are concepts of the ICRP and the NCRP. ORP stands for Optimization of Radiation Protection. The history of the ALARA concept is traced back to the Manhattan Project of World War-II that radiation exposures be kept at lowest possible level.

The greatest risk to the fetus of chromosomal abnormalities and subsequent mental retardation is between 8 and 15 weeks of pregnancy and examinations involving radiation to the fetus should be avoided during this period. For examinations which may involve rather heavy doses or radiation such as Barium enemas, pelvic or abdominal CT, the examination should be carried out during the first 10 days of the menstrual cycle to avoid irradiation any possible pregnancy. Avoiding repeat exposures by employing proper exposure factors, and maintaining a proper record of films are means to reduce the radiation dose.

"Optimization of protection" can be achieved by "optimization of the radiological procedure" so as to reduce radiation exposures to the minimum levels. This optimization is possible by good quality assurance and quality control. Factors which can contribute to dose reduction and quality assurance are, the use of high frequency three-phase generator equipment, use of high KV technique and low mAs (using the shortest exposure time), beam collimation using proper beam filtration, using an X-ray table top which allows high beam transmission, antiscatter grids, high speed films with rare earth screens, optimal film processing and largest possible source to image receptor distance (SID).

High frequency generators help in generating high KV for use in the "high KV and low mAs technique". The high KV beam has higher energy photons, which undergo a lesser degree of beam attenuation and greater penetration of the beam through the patient.

Therefore the tissue deposition of photon is reduced, and therefore reduces the radiation dose to the patient.

Tube current or mA determines the quantity of the photons which also contribute to the patient dose. Increased exposure time also contributes to an increased patient dose. Since patient exposure is determined by exposure rate and time, the use of high frequency generators which generate high KV beam will decrease the mAs required to produce diagnostically adequate X-rays and hence reduce radiation dose to the patient.

Beam filtration causes lower energy photons to be absorbed by the filters thus increase the mean energy of the beam and its penetrating power and hence decrease the patient dose. Field of view (FOV) which is the size of the irradiated area, directly effects the patient dose. Beam collimators control the FOV such, that only the diagnostically important area is irradiated. A good alignment between the field of the collimator and the radiation beam, reduces the possibility of beam cut of and beam overlap, thus reduces the chances of diagnostically inadequate exposures and prevents repeat exposures. The table top should be one which allows a high beam transmission which increases the quantity of diagnostically important photons reaching the film. A carbon fibre material is generally used for a high transmission table top. Antiscatter grids reduce scattered radiation reaching the film thus improving the quality of the resulting the radiograph and reducing chances of repeat exposures.

Correct exposure factors and technical considerations have a significant contribution towards patient shielding for CT examination as well. For a CT examination of the skull, correct gantry angulation and beam collimation significantly reduces radiation dose to the orbits, despite the proximity of these organs to the X-ray beam, whereas the converse is true if correct technical considerations are not adhered to.(Robinson *et al.*, 1997)

Triad of radiation protection actions comprise "time-distance-shielding". Reducing of exposure time, increasing distance from source, and shielding of patients and occupational workers have proven to be of great importance in protecting patients, personnel, and members of the public from the potential risks of radiation.

Time

The exposure time is related to radiation exposure and exposure rate (exposure per unit time) as follows:

$$\text{Exposure time} = \frac{\text{Exposure}}{\text{Exposure rate}}$$

Or

$$\text{Exposure} = \text{Exposure rate} \times \text{Time}$$

The algebraic expressions simply imply that if the exposure time is kept short, then the resulting dose to the individual is small.

Distance

The second radiation protection action relates to the distance between the source of radiation and the exposed individual. The exposure to the individual decrease inversely as the square of the distance. This is known as the inverse square law, which is stated mathematically as:

$$I \; a \; \frac{1}{d^2}$$

where I is the intensity of radiation and d is the distance between the radiation source and the exposed individual.

In mobile radiography, where there is not fixed protective control booth, the technologist should remain at least 2 m from the patient, the X-ray tube, and the primary beam during the exposure. In this respect, the ICRP (1982), as well as the NCRP (1989a), recommended that the length of the exposure cord on mobile radiographic units be at least 2 m long.

SHIELDING

The third radiation protection action relates to shielding. Shielding implies that certain materials (concrete, lead) attenuate radiation (reduce its intensity) when they are placed between the source of radiation and the exposed individual.

Four aspects of shielding:

1. X-ray tube shielding.
2. Room shielding:
   a. X-ray equipment room shielding.
   b. Patient waiting room shielding.
3. Personnel shielding.
4. Patient shielding (of organs not under investigation).

X-ray Tube Shielding (Source Shielding)

The X-ray tube housing is lined with thin sheets of lead because X-ray produced in the tube are scattered in all directions. This shielding is intended to protect both patients and personnel from leakage of radiation. Leakage radiation is that created at the X-ray tube anode but not emitted through the X-ray tube portal. Leakage radiation is transmitted through tube housing. Manufacturers of X-ray devices are required to shield the tube housing so as to limit the leakage radiation exposure rate to 0.1 Rhr^{-1} at 1 metre from the tube anode.[Simpkin *et al.*, 1998] AERB recommends a maximum allowable leakage radiation from tube housing not greater than 1 mGy per hour per 100 cm^2.

Room Shielding (Structural Shielding)

The lead lined walls of Radiology department are referred to as protective barriers because they are designed to protect individuals located outside the X-ray rooms from unwanted radiation. There are two types of protective barriers.

a. **Primary Barrier:** is one which is directly struck by the primary or the useful beam.

b. **Secondary Barrier:** is one which is exposed to secondary radiation either by leakage from X-ray tube or by scattered radiation from the patient.
c. **Control Area:** is defined as the area routinely occupied by radiation workers who are exposed to an occupational dose. For control area, the shielding should be such that it reduces exposure in that area to <26 mC/kg/week.
d. **Uncontrolled Areas:** are those areas which are not occupied by occupational workers. For these areas, the shielding should reduce the exposure rate to <2.6 mC/kg/week.(Seeram *et al.*, 1997)

X-ray Examination Room Shielding

Rooms housing diagnostic X-ray units and related equipment are located as far away as feasible from areas of high occupancy and general traffic, such as maternity and paediatric wards and other departments of the hospital that are not directly related to radiation and its use. The room housing of an X-ray unit is not less than 18 m^2 for general purpose radiography and conventional fluoroscopy equipment. In case, the installation is located in a residential complex, it is ensured that (i) walls of the X-ray room on which primary X-ray beam falls is not less than 35 cm thick brick or equivalent, (ii) walls of the X-ray room on which scattered X-rays fall is not less than 23 cm thick brick or equivalent, (iii) there is a shielding equivalent to at least 23 cm thick brick or 1.7 mm lead in front or the doors and windows of the X-ray room to protect the adjacent areas, either used by general public or not under possession of the owner of the X-ray room. Unshielded openings in an X-ray room for ventilation or natural light, are located above a height of 2 m from the finished level outside the X-ray room. Rooms housing fluoroscopy equipment are so designed that adequate darkness can be achieved conveniently, when desired, in the room.

Patient Waiting Area

Patient waiting areas are provided outside the X-ray room. A suitable warning signal such as red light and a warning playcard is provided at a conspicuous place outside the X-ray room and kept 'ON' when the unit is in use to warn the persons not connected with the particular examination from entering the room.

Shielding of the X-ray Control Room

The control room of X-ray equipment is a secondary protective barrier which has two important aspects:

a. The walls and viewing window of the control booth, which should have lead equivalents of 1.5 mm.

b. The location of control booth, which should not be located where the primary beam falls directly, and the radiation should be scattered twice before entering the booth.(Seeram *et al.*, 1997)

The control panel of diagnostic X-ray equipment operating at 125 kVp or above is installed in a separate room located outside but contiguous to the X-ray room and provided with appropriate shielding, direct viewing and oral communication facilities between the operator and the patient. In case of X-ray equipment operating upto 125 kVp, the control panel can be located in the X-ray room. AERB recommends that the distance between control panel and X-ray unit/chest stand should not be less than 3 m for general purpose fixed X-ray equipment.

The highly collimated X-ray beam in CT results in markedly non-uniform distribution of absorbed dose perpendicular to the tomographic plane during the CT exposure. Therefore the size of the CT room housing the gantry of the CT unit as recommended by AERB should not be less than 25 m^2.

Personnel Shielding

Shielding of occupational workers can be achieved by following methods:

a. Personnel should remain in the radiation environment only when necessary (stay behind the control booth, or leave the room when practical).

b. The distance between the personnel and the patient should be maximized when practical as the intensity of radiation decreases as the square of distance (inverse square law).

c. Shielding apparel should be used as and when necessary which comprise lead aprons, eye glasses with side shields, hand gloves and thyroid shields.

Lead aprons are shielding apparel recommended for use by radiation workers. These are classified as a secondary barrier to the effects of ionizing radiation. These aprons protect an individual only from secondary (scattered) radiation, not the primary beam. The thickness of lead in the protective apparel determines the protection it provides. It is known that 0.25 mm lead thickness attenuates 66% of the beam at 75 kVp and 1 mm attenuates 99% of the beam at same kVp. For general purpose radiography, the minimum thickness of lead equivalent in the protective apparel should be 0.5 mm. Women radiation workers should wear a customized lead apron that reaches below mid thigh level and wraps completely around the pelvis. This would eliminate an accidental exposure to a conceptus.(Wagner *et al.*, 1982)

Lead aprons should not be abused, such as by dropping them on the floor, piling them in a heap or improperly draping them over the back of a chair. Because all of these actions can cause internal fracturing of the lead, they may compromise the apron's protective ability. When not in use, all protective apparel should be hung on properly designed racks protective apparel also should be radiographed for defects such as internal cracks and tears at least once in a year.(Shymko MJ, 1998)

Other protective apparel includes eyeglasses with side shields, thyroid shields and gloves. The minimum protective lead equivalents in hand gloves and thyroid shields should be 0.5 mm.

AERB Guidelines for Personal Protection

The protective barrier between the operator and X-ray tube should have a minimum lead equivalence of 1.5 mm protective aprons and gloves should have a minimum lead equivalence of 0.25 mm, and gonadal shields should have a minimum lead equivalence of 0.5 mm. Any additional radiation protection devices which would be necessary for specialized radiological investigations should have a minimum of 0.5 mm lead equivalence.

Patient Shielding

It has been recommended that the thyroid, breast and gonads be shielded, to protect these organs especially in children and young adults. In gonadal shielding, a lead apron is placed appropriately on the patient to protect the gonads from primary beam radiation exposure. A lead bib and collar worn over the patient's neck and thorax have been documented to effectively shield radiosensitive organs like the thyroid and the breast, and are therefore recommended for routine use in dental X-rays and head CT examinations.(Beacomfield *et al.*, 1998)

Radiation in the CT Suite

CT accounts for less than 50% of all X-ray examinations, it contributes upto 40% of the collective dose from diagnostic radiology. CT scanners have scattered radiation levels that may prove hazardous. The dose unit used in CT is the computed tomography dose index "CTDI". This measurement is defined in relation to the radiation field delivered at a specific point (x, y) by the CT scanner. CTDI is usually expressed in terms of absorbed dose to tissue (D_{tissue}) is related to absorbed dose to air (D_{air}) by a mathematical coefficient which has a value of about 1.06 and an error not greater than $\pm 1\%$. Such measurements are made using a special pencil ionization chamber or by a thermoluminescent dosimeter (TLD). Scattered radiation in a CT suite could be as high as 0.3 Gy/day. Additional thickness of 2.5 mm of lead or 162 mm of concrete to shield the front and rear reference points, so as to reduce the dose of 1 mGy/year.(Langer *et al.*, 1998)

Radiation Protection in CT Suite

Radiologists who work in CT fluoroscopy (CTF) should employ lead glasses, thyroid shields, lead aprons, lead gloves, and portable body radiation barriers. They should wear both internal and external radiation badges to monitor their exposure to scattered radiation during the procedures. This allows the radiation levels associated with CTF to be measured so that radiologists can be judicious in selecting CT technique settings and in minimizing the fluoroscopic time for each procedure. Radiation exposure to patient and staff during CTF can be controlled by employing low mA sittings, limiting imaging times, and employing appropriate radiation protection measures.(Nickoloff *et al.*, 2000)

Radiation Detection and Measurement

Radiation detection devices are the instruments used to measure radiation are called radiation dosimeters.

Methods of Detection

There are several methods of detecting radiation, and they are based on physical and chemical effects produced by radiation exposure. These methods are:

1. Ionization chamber.
2. Photographic effect.
3. Luminescence.
4. Scintillation.

Ionization: The ability of radiation to produce ionization in air is the basis for radiation detection by the ionization chamber. It consists of an electrode positioned in the middle of a cylinder that contains gas. When X-rays enter the chamber, they ionize the gas to gram negative ions (electrons) and positive ions (positrons). The electrons are collected by the positively changed rod, while the positive ions are attracted to the negatively charged wall of the cylinder. The resulting small current from the chamber is subsequently amplified and measured. The strength of the current is proportional to the radiation intensity.

Photographic Effect: The photographic effect, which refers to the ability of radiation to blacken photographic films, is the basis of detectors that use film.

Luminescence: Luminescence describes the property by which certain materials emit light when stimulated by a physiological process, a chemical or electrical action, or by heat. When radiation strikes these materials, the electrons are raised to higher orbital levels. When they fall back to their original orbital level, light is emitted. The amount of light emitted is proportional to the radiation intensity. Lithium fluoride, for example, will emit light when stimulated by heat. This is the fundamental basis of thermoluminescence dosimetry (TLD), a method used to measure exposure to patients and personnel.

Scintillation: Scintillation refers to a flash of light. It is a property of certain crystals such as sodium iodide and cesium iodide to absorb radiation and convert it to light. This light is then directed to a photomultiplier tube, which then converts the light into an electrical pulse. The size of the pulse is proportional to the light intensity, which then converts the light into an electrical pulse. The size of the pulse is proportional to the light intensity, which is in turn proportional to the energy of the radiation.

Personnel Dosimetry

Personnel dosimetry to the monitoring of individuals who are exposed to radiation during the course of their work. Personnel dosimetry policies need to be in place for all occupationally exposed individuals. Proper care include not irradiating the dosimeter except during occupational exposure and ensuring proper environmental conditions.

Monitoring is accomplished through the use of personnel dosimeters such as the pocket dosimeter, the film badge or the thermoluminescent dosimeter. The radiation measurement is a time-integrated dose, i.e., the dose summed over a period of time, usually about 3 months. The dose is subsequently stated as an estimate of the effective dose equivalent to the whole body in mSv for the reporting period. Dosimeters used for personnel monitoring have dose measurement limit of 0.1-0.2 mSv (10-20 mrem).

Pocket Dosimeter

The pocket dosimeter monitors dose to personnel. It consists of an ionization chamber with an eyepiece and a transparent scale, as well as a hollow charging rod and a fixed and a movable fiber. When X-rays enter the dosimeter, ionization causes the fibers to lose their charges and, as a result, the movable fiber moves closer to the fixed fiber. The movable fiber provides and estimates gamma or X-ray dose rate.

Film Badge Monitoring

These badges use small X-ray films sandwiched between several filters to help detect radiation. Film badges are inexpensive, easy to use, and easy to process. Although they are useful for detecting radiation at or above 0.1 mSv (10 mrem), they are not sensitive enough to capture lower levels of radiation. Their susceptibility to fogging caused by high temperature and light means that they cannot and should not be worn for longer than a 4-week period at a stretch. Another major drawback to film badge monitoring is that it is an enormous task to chemically process a large number of small films and subsequently compare each to some standard test film. In India, film badges have recently been replaced by TLD badges.

Thermoluminescent Dosimetry (TLD) Monitoring

The limitations of the film badge are overcome by the thermoluminescent dosimeter (TLD). Thermoluminescence is the property of certain materials to emit light when they are stimulated by heat. Materials such as lithium fluoride (LiF), lithium borate ($Li_2B_4O_7$), calcium fluoride (CaF_2), and calcium sulfate ($CaSO_4$) have been used to make TLDs.

When an LiF crystal is exposed to radiation, a few electrons become trapped in higher energy levels. For these electrons to return to their normal energy levels, the LiF crystal must be heated. As the electrons return to their stable state, light is emitted because of the energy difference between two orbital levels. The amount of light emitted is measured (by a photomultiplier tube) and it is proportional to the radiation dose.

The measurement of radiation from a TLD is a two-step procedure. In step 1, the TLD is exposed to the radiation. In step 2, the LiF crystal is placed in a TLD analyzer, where it is exposed to heat. As the crystal is exposed to increasing temperatures, light is emitted. When the intensity of light is plotted as a function of the temperature, a glow curve results. The glow curve can be used to find out how much radiation energy is received by the crystal because the highest peak and the area under the curve are proportional to the energy of the radiation.

Whereas the TLD can measure exposures to individuals as low as 1.3 μC.kg (5 mR), the pocket dosimeter can measure upto 50 μC/kg (200 mR). The film badge, however, cannot measure exposure <2.6 μC/kg (10 mR). TLDs can withstand a certain degree of heat, humidity and pressure; their crystals are reusable; and instantaneous readings are possible if the department has a TLD analyzer. The greatest disadvantage of a TLD is its cost.

Wearing the Dosimeter

a. **During Radiography**

During radiography (when no protective lead apron is worn), the personnel dosimeter is worn at one of two regions:

1. On the trunk of the body at the level of the waist, on the anterior side of the individual.

OR

2. On the upper chest region at the level of the collar area on the anterior surface of the individual.

b. **During Fluoroscopy**

During fluoroscopy a protective apron should always be worn. Ideally two dosimeters should be worn by radiation personnel.

One at the collar level outside the lead apron and the other at the trunk level underneath the lead apron.

The one at the collar level gives an accurate estimate of the radiation dose to the unprotected regions of head and neck. The dosimeter worn underneath the lead apron at the trunk level provides an accurate estimate of the radiation to the protected organs. If only one dosimeter is worn, it must be worn at the collar outside the lead apron, because, the neck receives 10-20 times more radiation than the trunk which is protected by lead.

Radiation Protection Survey Programme

The responsibility for establishing a radiation protection programme rests with the hospital administration/owners of the X-ray facility. Radiation Safety Committee (RSC), Radiation Safety Officer (RSO) recommended by NCRP that the RSC should comprise a radiologist, a medical physicist, a nuclear medicine personnel, a senior nurse and an internist. It is the duty of RSC to perform a regular radiation protection survey. This survey has 5 phases which are:

1. **Investigation:** To obtain information regarding layout of the department, workload, personnel monitoring and records.
2. **Inspection:** Each diagnostic installation in the department is examined for its protection status with respect to its operating factors, control booth and availability of protection devices.
3. **Measurement:** Measurements are conducted on exposure factors. In addition scattered radiation and patient dose measurements in radiography and fluoroscopy are performed.
4. **Evaluation:** The radiation protection status of the department is evaluated by examination of records, equipment working, status of protective clothing and the radiation doses obtained from phase 3.

5. **Recommendations:** A report is prepared on the protection status of the department and the problem areas if any identified, for which recommendations are made regarding corrective measures.

Surveillance of Radiation Workers

AERB has recommended regular medical examination of radiation workers to assess their protection status as per the following guidelines:

"Every radiation worker prior to commencing radiation work and at subsequent intervals not exceeding 12 months shall be subjected to the following medical examinations:

1. X-ray examination of chest.
2. All general laboratory investigations such as examination of blood, urine and stool.
3. Special investigations such as examination of skin, hands, fingers, nails and eyes."

Radiation Safety Officer

NCRP has provided a brief description of the relevant qualifications and duties of an RSO. Every department should have an RSO. This officer should be an individual with extensive training and education in areas such as radiation protection, radiation physics, radiation biology, instrumentation, dosimetry and shielding design.

	Occupational workers			**Public**
	Limit	*Annual equivalents*	*Limit*	*Annual equivalents*
ICRP	20 mgSv/yr over 5 years	20 mSv	1 mSv/yr over 5 years	1 mSv
NCRP	Cumulative dose = Age in yrs × 10 mSv	50 mSv period	5 mSv for 5 years	1 mSv
AERB	100 mSv for 5 years period	30 mSv	1 mSv/yr for 5 years	1 mSv

AERB has specified duties of the RSO which include assisting the employer in meeting the relevant regulatory requirements applicable to his/her X-ray installation. He/she shall implement all radiation surveillance measures, conduct periodic radiation protection surveys, maintain proper records of periodic quality assurance tests, and personnel doses, instruct all workers on relevant safety measures, educate and train new entrants, and take local measures, including issuance of clear administrative instructions of writing, to deal with radiation emergencies. The RSO should also ensure that all radiation measuring and monitoring instruments in his/her custody are properly calibrated and maintained in good condition. The duties also include maintaining a record of all radiation surveys performed, deficiencies observed and remedial actions taken.

Recommended Dose Limits for Radiation Workers and General Public

	Dose limits to skin, hands, feet (mSv/yr)	*Dose limits to lens of eye (mSv/yr)*
ICRP	500	150
NCRP	500	150
AERB	500	150

Recommended Dose Limits to Pregnant Women

The recommendations:

1. **ICRP:** In pregnant females, a supplementary equivalent dose limit of 2 mSv applied to the surface of her lower abdomen for the remainder of her pregnancy.
2. **NCRP:** Recommends dose limit 0.5 mSv per month for the embryo/fetus for occupational pregnant workers.
3. **AERB:** Recommends that once pregnancy is established the equivalent to surface of pregnant woman's abdomen should not exceed 2 mSv for the remainder of the pregnancy.

Estimated fetal exposure for various diagnostic imaging methods

Examination type	*Estimated fetal dose per examination (rad)**	*Estimated fetal dose per examination (m gray/m Sv)**	*Number of examinations required for a cumulative 5-rad (0.05 gray) dose*
Plain films			
Skull	0.004	0.04	1,250
Chest (two views)	0.00007	0.0007	71,429
Mammogram	0.002	0.02	250
Lumbosacral spine	0.359	3.59	13
Pelvis	0.040	0.40	125
CT scans (slice thickness: 10 mm)			
Head (10 slices)	<0.050	<0.50	>100
Abdomen (10 slices)	<0.100	<1.0	>50
Fluoroscopic studies			
Upper GI series	0.56	5.6	89
Nuclear medicine studies			
Most studies using technetium (99m Tc)	<0.500	<5.00	>10
Environmental sources			
(For comparison) Environmental background radiation (cumulative dose over nine months)	0.100	1.00	N/A

Minimum Protection Requirement for a Safe Diagnostic Unit

i. Each diagnostic unit installation should have a minimum area of about 225 sq.ft.

ii. A red light should be placed outside the room, to stop and prevent any one entering the room when, an X-ray is in progress.

iii. Walls of an X-ray should have adequate thickness to absorb and stop the radiation produced.

iv. Doors of an X-ray room should be adequately lead-lined.

v. More than one X-ray examination should not be performed simultaneously in one room and hence installation of more than one unit in a single room should be avoided.

vi. No member of the staff must hold children or infirm patients for radiography. A relative or escort, who is a non-radiation worker should be asked to do this work and should be provided with radiation protection means, like lead aprons and gloves.

vii. In all diagnostic procedures, particular attention must be given to the protection of gonads of both patients and others.

viii. Lead rubber aprons and lead rubber gloves should be used during screening of the patient.

ix. The aprons and gloves should be checked periodically for their wear and tear (cracks).

x. In case of number of special investigations, where radiation dose is heavy, the person on duty should perform a rotational duty to be preferably changed/rotated weekly.

xi. A series of X-ray investigations should not be done on same patient consecutively, especially for persons below age of 40 years. In such patients genetic damage can be significant.

METHODS OF PROTECTION

The protection is achieved by ensuring that:

1. The installation is adequate.
2. Proper protection is adequate.
3. The equipment used is satisfactory as per quality and radiation protection norms.
4. The work practices followed are satisfactory.

Diagnostic X-ray Installation Recommendations

Use or Protective Devices

Protective Barrier:

In case of diagnostic tubes operating at 150 kv and above, the control panel should be located in a separate room and the technician should position himself inside the control room whenever the tube is energized. In case of diagnostic tubes operating at 100 kV, the control panel should be located either in a separate room or behind a mobile protective barrier of 1.5 mm lead equivalence or a partition wall with a viewing window of lead glass of 1.5 mm lead equivalence as far away as possible but not less 2 meter from the tube should be installed. The technician should position himself behind the protective shielding during each exposure. If the unit is located in a separate room the means of communication between the patient and operator at the control panel should be provided.

In case of radiography, the vertical cassette holder (chest stand), should have a backing of at least 1.5 mm thick lead.

The dose to gonads of the patients should be reduced by using gonad shields. Bucky should be covered by shielding devices having lead equivalence of not less than 0.5 mm.

In case of fluoroscopy machines, the shutter control should be so shielded as to provide adequate protection for hands of lead equivalence of 1.5 mm lead up to 70 kV and 2 mm between 70 kV and 100 kV. Above 100 kV, the thickness should be increased by 0.01 mm for each kV increase.

Work Practices

All steps should be taken to ensure that unnecessary exposures are not received by any person whether the radiation worker himself, the patient or public at large. Hence all the protective devices must be used. All such measures should be adopted that the exposures are reduced. The protective devices should be regularly checked for their protection adequacy, the beam limiting diaphragm should be checked periodically to ensure that radiation and light beam fields coincide and they define the beam correctly. It should also be ensured periodically that the primary beam does not escape through the diaphragm due to wear and tear or bad condition of the X-ray tube itself.

To avoid necessary exposures it should be ensured that the red light warning signal is made 'on' before giving the exposures. There should not be any person other than those required for the examination in the X-ray room.

Special care should be taken for X-ray examination of persons of reproductive age specially woman. The X-ray examination of pelvis and abdomen of a lady of reproductive group should be done during first ten days from the first day of the menstrual period. The X-ray examination of pregnant lady must be avoided specially when they are in 8-15 week period. If the exposures are given during this period, there are chances of mental retardation.

Radiation worker should not hold children or infant patients. In unavoidable cases, if they have to hold or any of the relative holds, the protective apron must be worn and he or she should stand by the side of patient.

Proper distance between focus to the patient or cassette should be kept so that the divergence of the beam in passing through the body is minimum and the dose to the patient is within limits. For example in fluoroscopy, the patient to focus distance should not be less than 45 cm, in radiography, the distance between patient and cassette should not be less than 40 inches. In case of screening palpation should not be done by bare or even gloved hands. A palpation spoon should be used. It may be noted that gloves or aprons offer protection against secondary radiation and not against primary radiation.

UNIT FOR STUDY OF RADIATION

Absorbed Dose:

Absorbed dose is a term used for purpose of radiation protection and assess the dose or risk to human in general. Absorbed dose is the amount of radiation absorbed in an organ or tissue (amount of radiation energy that has been left in cells, tissue or an organ). Absorbed dose is usually defined as energy deposited (Joule) per unit of mass.

Roentgen:

Roentgen is "that amount of X, or gamma radiation that the associated corpuscular emission, per 0.001293 gram of air, produces in air ions carrying one electrostatic unit of charge of either sign".

Roentgen is amount of radiation incident upon the material.

$1R = 2.58 \times 10^{-4}$ coulomb/Kg of air.

Roentgen (R) is used to describe radiation exposure. The term describes the amount of ionization in air. In the International system of units, the coulomb/Kg (CKg^{-1}) describes radiation exposure.

Curie:

Curie (Ci) is the traditional unit used to describe the amount of radioactive material present or strength of the source.

Becquerel:

Becquerel (Bq) is the unit in the International system of unit to replace the Curie. It is based upon the radioactive decay rate of the radionucleide. One Bq is equal to one disintegration per sec (DPS). The most common activity level used in laboratory is the megabecquerel (MBq). A megabecquerel is one million Bq and equal to 22 microcurie (μci), 37 gigabecquerel (GBq) is equal to one Curie.

Gray:

Dr. L. H. Gray, after whom the new unit is named, made fundamental contribution to radiation dosemetry. In June 1975 International committee on weight and measures adopted the gray (Gy) as standard International unit of absorbed dose.

1 gray = 1 Joule / Kg = 100 rad.

RAD:

1 rad = 100 ergs per gram (amount of energy absorbed as the result of the exposure).

OR

1 rad = 0.01 Gy = 0.01 J / Kg.

REM:

Rem is traditional unit used to describe equivalent or effective radiation dose.

Sievert:

Sv is the unit in the international system of units to describe equivalent or effective radiation dose.

1 Sv = 100 rem.

It is a unit that is the product of energy absorbed in human tissue and the quality of radiation being absorbed (ability of the radiation to cause damage).

1 Gy = 100 rad

1 mGy = 100 mrad

1 Sv = 100 rem

1 mSv = 100 mrem

Tissue Weighting Factor:

A number assigned to various tissues taking in account, the tissue's sensitivity to radiation, i.e., how likely it is that the tissue will be affected by radiation dose it receives.

Radiation Weighting Factor:

Radiation weighting factor are dimensionsless factors developed for radiation protection to assess health risk from radiation dose, taking into account the biological effectiveness of different types of radiation.

Threshold Erethema Dose:

T.E.D. is amount of radiation which would produce a just perceptible reddening of the skin in 80% of those exposed.

INDEX

A

Abdomen 78

Acquisition of radiograph 28

Anatomical terminology 35

Ankle joint 101

Antegrade pyelography 177

Antero-posterior view for

- liver 82
- pregnancy 82
- spleen 82

Arteriography and angiocardiography 193

Arthrography 200

Ascending urethrography in male 184

B

Barium

- enema 152
- meal 143

Biliary tract and pancreas 161

Biological effects of radiation 285

Bladder 290

Burhenne technique 169

C

Calcaneum 107

Cassette 26

Central nervous system 200

Cervicodorsal spine 61

Chest 66

Chronic radiation effects 288

Classification of radiation injury 287

Computed tomography 218

Contrast medium for MRI 140

Contrast of the film 12

Conventional versus low-osmolar contrast media 129

Coccyx 116

Craniocaudal view 266

CT system 223

Curie Temperature 208

Curve characteristic 19

D

Dacryocystography 201

Dark-room artefacts 32

Dark-room chemistry 29

Data acquisition systems 223
DEXA 269, 271
Density 9
Digestive tract 290
Digital Radiography 25
Digital subtraction angiography 274
Diaphragm 77
Dorsolumbar vertebrae 62

E

Echoplanar imaging 249
Elbow joint anteroposterior view 87
Elbow joint lateral view 88
Electronic transducer 213
Endoluminal contrast agents 258
Equipments for an angiography room 194
ERCP 166
Evaluation criteria 263
Excretory urography 173
Eye 290

F

Femur 95
Film fogs 31
Fistulogram 160
Focussed transducer 210
Foot 103
Forearm anteroposterior (AP) view 89
Forearm lateral view 89
Foreign body esophagus 76
Four slice design 227
Fourth generation system 224

G

Gadodiamide 140
Gadolinium 251
Gastrointestinal tract 141
Gynaecography 191

H

Hand lateral view 91
Hand
- anterior oblique view 91
- anteroposterior (AP) view 90

Hard X-ray 3
Harmful effects of radiation 278
Head and neck 43
Heart and blood vessels 289
Heart and great vessels 73
Hemopoietic system 290
Hip joint 111
Hysterosalpingography 189

I

Instant barium enema 156
Intensifying screen 27
Interaction of radiation with matter 285
Intravascular contrast media 126

K

Knee joint 97

L

Latitude and sensitivity 22
Leg 100

Ligands/chelates 252
Loopogram 160
Lordotic view 69
Lower extremity 95
Lower ribs 71
Lumbar vertebrae 63
Lumbosacral vertebrae 64
Luminescence 309
Lung 290
Lymph gland and lymphatics 198

M

Magnetic resonance imaging 240
Magnetisation transfer contrast 249
Mammography 259
Maximum permissible dose 33
Mechanical transducer 212
Mechanism of radiation induced cancer 292
Mentic view 54
Micturating cystourethrogram 182
MLO view 264
MR angiography 255
Multislice spiral CT 227

N

Nephrolithotomy 186
Nephrostomy 178
Non-ionic contrast medium 138

O

Oblique 38
Omniscan 140
Osteoporosis and osteopenia 269
Other radiation induced cancers 292

P

Patella 98
Pathology of radiation injury 286
Patient shielding 307
Pelvis 110
Percutaneous nephrostomy 178, 186
Personnel dosimetry 309
PET-CT 235
Pharmacokinetics 252
Pharynx and larynx 75
Piezoelectric crystals 207
Pocket dosimeter 310
Positioning technique 262
Positioning terminology 35
Posterior oblique 39
Pregnant radiation worker 296
Projection terminology 37
Properties of X-rays 2
Pulse sequences 247

R

Radiation hazards 284
Radiation measurements 279
Radiographic quality 7
Radiological procedures including contrast media 121
Reducing scattered radiation 15
Renal cyst puncture 176
Replenisher 30
Reproductive system 188

Retrograde pyelogram 180
Retroperitoneal structures 81
Risk estimates for radiation induced cancer 292
Rotating anode 7

S

Sacroiliac joint 117
Sacrum 114
Schuller's view 47
Scintillation 309
Screen speed 27
Shortening of life span 291
Sialography 202
Sinogram 159
Skin 289
Small bowel enema 149
Soft X-ray 4
Somatic stochastic effects 291
Spine or vertebral column 57
Spiral/helical computed tomography 226
Stationary anode 5
Stenver's view 48
Sternum 71
Submandibular gland 203

T

T-tube cholangiography 162
Technical aspect 205
Temporomandibular joint 54
Testis and ovaries 290
Therapeutic gastrografin enema 158
Thermoluminescent dosimetry 310
Third generation system 224
Tissue weighting factor 320
Toes 105
TOF MR angiography 256
Towne's view 45
Transducers 207
Trazogastro 136
Types of films 23
Types of grids 17

U

Ultrasonography 205
Upper extremity 83
Urinary tract 81, 171

V

Venography 196
Vesiculography 191

W

Wrist: Lateral view 94
Wrist: Posteroanterior view 93

X

X-rays 1